A Moment
of Grace

Patrick Dillon

EBURY
PRESS

1 3 5 7 9 10 8 6 4 2

This edition published in 2019 by Ebury Press, an imprint of Ebury Publishing

20 Vauxhall Bridge Road
London SW1V 2SA

Ebury Press is part of the Penguin Random House group of companies
whose addresses can be found at global.penguinrandomhouse.com

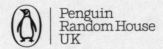

Penguin
Random House
UK

First published by Ebury Press in 2018
This edition published in 2019

www.penguin.co.uk

A CIP catalogue record for this book is available from the British Library

ISBN 9781785038471

Printed and bound in Great Britain by Clays Ltd, Elcograf S.p.A.

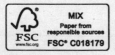

MIX
Paper from
responsible sources
FSC
www.fsc.org
FSC® C018179

Penguin Random House is committed to a sustainable
future for our business, our readers and our planet.
This book is made from Forest Stewardship Council®
certified paper.

NICOLA THOROLD

1965 – 2016

1

This is the story of my wife's death from leukaemia. It isn't a sad book. In our last year together we were more happy, in some ways, than we've ever been. She was fifty-one. Our two children were adults by the time Nicola died.

Nicola worked at the Roundhouse in London's Chalk Farm. She produced shows there – theatre, circus and dance. A few months before she fell ill, she put on Monteverdi's *L'Orfeo* in partnership with the Royal Opera House. On the opening night we stood talking in the foyer as the audience flowed up the stairs. Nicola wasn't most people's idea of a theatre producer: she wasn't flamboyant or extrovert, she was genuine, natural and unaffected. Her parents, Anne and Peter, were there. We talked to friends we'd known for years; to people from the production team; to the designer who'd worked on the show. Talk rose up between the old brick walls of the Roundhouse, filled the bar, diffused above us; next door we could hear the orchestra tuning up. Nicola glowed. She was doing what she cared for most, surrounded by the people she loved. She was in her world.

Inside the auditorium, lights winked on the roof of the Roundhouse, high above us, and the row of iron columns at our backs. I could tell Nicola was nervous and squeezed her hand in encouragement. How many shows had we been to together? I'd never thought of counting. We'd be going to them, I imagined, for as long as we both lived – until we were old together, still doing the things we most loved.

The lights dimmed. We heard the familiar rustle of the audience hushing as attention focused on the stage. The music began. They'd cast young singers in the leading roles. I'd seen the opera before, so I knew the story of the poet who goes to hell to retrieve his dead wife, Eurydice, and persuades Hades to let him return her to the light – so long as he doesn't look back. I didn't feel any premonition. Four months later, Nicola would be diagnosed with leukaemia, and a year after that she would be dead; but I didn't know, then, that I would have to set out on my own journey to recover her – that I, too, would find myself in a dark place, the road lost, searching for the gates of hell.

There was a wonderful party afterwards. We took the tube home. *L'Orfeo* wasn't the last show we went to. We spent Easter in France, and had a weekend in Madrid to celebrate

Nicola's fiftieth birthday. We had no warning of what was to come when our GP rang me at home, one Friday afternoon at the end of May.

'Mr Dillon?'

'Yes.'

'We're trying to get hold of your wife, Nicola Thorold.'

She'd been to the surgery that morning. In the last couple of weeks bruises had appeared on her legs, as if she'd knocked herself. Before that she'd had a virus, but she seemed to have shaken it off by the time we went to Madrid. Not quite herself, she managed the museums nonetheless: Goya and Velázquez. We found a blue-tiled restaurant, cool and high-ceilinged, and ate grilled shrimp and salad dressed with anchovies; she took rests in the afternoon. And then the bruises started to appear.

She ignored them until I bullied her into visiting the doctor.

'He took a blood test,' Nicola said when I called her late morning. She didn't sound worried. 'He said they'd get the results quickly.'

That haste was the only warning note, looking back. But we didn't hear it. I'd just left my job. As we spoke I was standing outside my old office, exhilarated. I was due to start at a new architects' practice on Monday. That evening we would celebrate freedom.

But the evening didn't arrive.

'We need to speak to her urgently, Mr Dillon. Do you have any way to get hold of her?'

'I can try her mobile.'

'She isn't answering.'

'What's it about?'

'I can't tell you that, Mr Dillon, but this is important. It's essential we see her before the weekend.'

'I'll try to get hold of her.'

My voice sounded unnaturally calm, even to myself. I was always good in a crisis, and this was already a crisis. As I put the phone down I knew this story had started. The GP's call was the first banging of a shutter, heralding a storm; the water slicking back along the harbour wall; the ground's tremor before an earthquake. Something was wrong.

Nicola's phone bleeped into a void, rhythmic and weak like the throb of a pulse, or a buoy flashing at sea to warn of danger. I tapped my finger on the desk to calm myself.

'Hello?' Her voice sounded normal.

'*Cara*.' My name for her. 'The doctor telephoned ...'

'I know, I got their message. I'm on the way home.'

'Did they say what it's about?'

'No.'

We both sounded calm. This, it was already agreed between us, was how we were going to handle the crisis – whatever it was. We knew each other. We'd been together

4

nearly thirty years. Whatever happened, we would be strong together.

'Shall I meet you at the surgery?'

'On the corner outside.'

I have her texts still. *Crossing Bridge* at 16.45 that Friday afternoon; at 16.47, *I'll meet you at Wincott Street*. I stood on the corner, waiting. Sometimes I feel as if I'm waiting there still – or as if, in that moment, life could have taken another turn. We could have met on the corner, happy, and gone to dinner to celebrate my new job; or met on the corner and gone home. I remember watching cars drone along Kennington Road. It was all so familiar: the newsagent, the parked cars and pelican crossing. But already everything was changing. Invisibly, our world was being packed away around me, like a funfair after the carnival. The places we loved, the habits we'd grown, were fading from sight, one by one. Our future was vanishing in fog.

We'd always been so lucky, until that Friday afternoon. And we knew how lucky we were. No landslides had carried us away; we'd suffered no catastrophes, bereavements or major illnesses. We came from happy, stable homes, loved our children, and earned enough to be comfortable. Time had rolled by in a dependable sequence, the years passing as solidly as stones in an ancient path, as if someone had gone that way before, to clear the track for us. Perhaps the only unusual thing about us was the depth of our love, a blissful, all-consuming love that had united us for twenty-eight years.

That, too, had begun on a street corner. Saturday, 14 November 1987, Nicola and I met on the pavement outside the Whitechapel Gallery. We'd already known each other for five years. I'd once stood in as a date for Nicola's high-school leaving dance – her boyfriend of the time was away. She wasn't quite beautiful then – it was later she became lovely – but she danced wonderfully, as if her grace was internal, revealed by music, and she was just waiting for the years to complete her. Nicola's eyes were a warm sea green. Her mouth was wide. When she smiled, her lips broke goofily along the line of her teeth; everyone loved her smile. Five years on, we were close friends. We'd both been in other relationships, but even so, there'd been moments along the way when we'd glimpsed what was to come. I stayed with her family in France one Easter. We were revising for exams, but escaped for a drive through woods to a castle nearby. Nicola had been going there since she was a child, when her parents bought the ramshackle old farmhouse in Aquitaine. It was her private place, revealed only to close friends. In driving me to the castle we both felt as if she was showing me something, pointing out a cleft in the horizon, a tower we would one day inhabit. Neither of us would have been surprised had someone predicted our future together, raising children, being happy.

So love had hovered around us, not quite landing, but then we found ourselves, in autumn 1987, with long-term relationships over. Nothing was said. Nicola came to spend a weekend in Suffolk, where I'd borrowed my sister's cottage on the river at Pin Mill. Perhaps I was showing her, in my turn, the places that I loved. Maybe we were displaying the treasures each could bring to our union, in a ritual as old and solemn as the meeting of families for an arranged marriage. Perhaps we were touring, in advance, the places where we would later build our life together.

The weekend after, the Whitechapel Gallery began a Cy Twombly retrospective. We wandered past the huge, textured canvases. They looked ancient, as if they had been rescued from pyramids or excavated from a rock face. There was writing on them: snatched words and phrases – *Apollo, Venus* – and looping figures, white on grey, that were almost writing. Our love and marriage would be an affair of words. *I think I might be falling in love with you* were the words Nicola spoke later, leaning back against my legs in the flat she shared with an old college friend. And in the years after that came endless conversations, lying in bed, walking home from the theatre, tramping through woods in France. Twenty-eight years of words scrawled on the walls of our lives. Birthdays and Christmases; the first words spoken in the morning and the last at night. And then, when she was in hospital and couldn't speak anymore, the texts we sent each other before sleeping: *Good night my darling husband. Good night my most perfect wife.*

I took her hand, as we sat on the floor of our friend's flat. Nicola never lacked for courage, and never lacked it later. If she wanted something, she wasn't scared to say so. She loved me, so she told me so. I remember the warmth of her lips when we kissed, the warmth of her fingers as they clutched mine. That night we slept in her tiny bedroom with a sloping ceiling and collapsible futon, and felt time surging into a future that felt inevitable: a future spent together.

And now, on a street corner in Kennington, time was collapsing in on us with a rush. We could almost feel it, like a cold breath on our faces. Normal life flowed by, but we were marooned within it; stuck fast, like a ship caught on a mudbank with the tide pouring out around it. People walked past, tired from the day, eyes intent on planning dinner, or the evening's phone calls; a bus hissed along the kerb; a dog tested its lead, snuffling the base of a wheelie bin. We were different: our future was gone.

We had nothing to go on except the doctor's call, but it was enough, already, to draw a curtain across the horizon. We'd booked a holiday in Greece in June, three weeks off. *We need to see her before the weekend.* Did that sound like the sort of thing that might be over in three weeks? Probably not. The grand recalibration of our lives was already under way. This book is the story of a star imploding in space, collapsing in on itself under forces too massive, too natural to resist; making no noise; an implosion so embedded in time as to be neither quick nor slow, because it makes its own time around it; because its rush is the thrum of time draining away, and the sudden darkness – the ensuing black hole – is time's end.

'Did they say anything on the phone?'

'No, just urgent.'

Nicola's face looked pointed and sharp. She was afraid, I knew, but determined not to show it. She was still wearing her work clothes. They'd be balled up, later, in a bag by her hospital bed and I'd take them home. She looked beautiful, two weeks before her hair went and the chemicals seared her flesh back to the bone. She looked beautiful afterwards.

We had one thing on our side, although we didn't know it then. It was magic of the most potent sort: we'd never taken one another for granted. That knowledge would strengthen us in the thirteen months we had left. It would strengthen us as Nicola's physical strength failed and her horizons narrowed. It would strengthen us even when she lay in intensive care in her last weeks, with machines winking in rows around her – blood pressure, temperature – and an oxygen tube whistling in her throat; as Chris or Anne-Marie, one of the nurses we got to know so well, deftly snapped another syringe of Fentanyl into the rack by her bed; as I held her hand under the sheet. We were never complacent about happiness. It was our blessing, not something to which we felt entitled.

Neither of us knew the GP, a locum, perhaps, or someone new. I've never seen him since, the man who pronounced my wife's death sentence.

'What exactly is wrong?'

'The consultants will want to talk to you about it.'

'It would be helpful to have some idea. Of course we're worrying.'

There were some books on his desk and a tired computer keyboard. It was the end of his day. Nicola sat up very straight, chin high. There was a focused look in her eyes. She was always so brave and matter-of-fact; a stoic, never one to sink her head in her hands.

The doctor didn't know which of us to look at, so he told me: 'They think ... they're fairly certain ... it's a leukaemia.'

We'd reached that moment from the movies; or from one of those wakeful nights when life veers off its tracks into imagined narratives of tragedy and disaster. But fiction and nightmare provide a kind of insulation; this was real.

I took it in. I didn't take it in. I looked at Nicola, who nodded at the doctor, absorbed not in herself, but in the conversation we were having with him. And something odd happened. In my own mind, like a shrill tinnitus behind the sound of their voices, came the thought, *This is just as one imagined.* It would be with me for the next thirteen months, that voice, until she died. The inner commentator; the detached part of oneself – detached even as one's ship ran onto the rocks, as the house burned – who watched and processed, recording the deterioration of our lives even as thermometer and oxygen probe tracked the decline of Nicola's body. *Just as one imagined* – and then, like the pad of a foot on the path behind us, fell the louder, nearer sound of what was actually happening: Nicola had cancer.

Our remaining time together would always carry that reverberation: our story, and the telling of our story a split-second behind it, like the echo in a church. Later on the ICU doctors would measure the slow failure of Nicola's body in the green-figured screens over which they pored so intently, concern and intelligence plaited on faces that gauged death's approach. And we too, in the next thirteen months, would learn to sense and measure each quivering emotion, to parse out the finest nuances of love and fear. The air was already rushing out through our lives, like a balloon deflating. I could feel its vibration under my fingertips. Perhaps capturing it felt like a way of slowing the rush. I was trying to tame shock through narrative, perhaps trying to turn what was happening to us into something that others might understand – which, I suppose, is why I'm writing this book.

The doctor was apologetic. Bad news on a Friday afternoon. To him, foot soldier in the NHS ranks, the duties of the firing line.

'I need to go home and get some things,' Nicola said. Only I could hear the nervousness in her voice.

And it was then we realised how close death was. 'No,' the doctor said. 'You really have to go to A&E straightaway.' His voice quivered. 'Right now, please. Now.'

He rang them. His phone call was the leper's bell, clearing the way ahead. One imagined alarms ringing down hospital corridors, beds made, nurses washing their fingers under a silver thread of water, as if Nicola's death was a ritual already begun. We were marked out, different even now from the old women dozing in the GP's waiting room as we went out, from the two receptionists gossiping behind the counter, from the commuter cycling home down Lambeth Bridge Road.

We walked side by side, not talking. We carried a burden no one else could see, a knowledge no one shared.

'Someone at work was diagnosed with leukaemia,' I said, filling the silence. 'There are different kinds of leukaemia, he said. His isn't terminal, it's just something he lives with. It's fine.'

'Of course it's going to be fine.'

Our instinct was to make this feel normal – whatever it was. The world had been knocked off its pole; we needed to put it back. Bad news need not be so bad. There was always a way ahead. Normality was our greatest wealth, and we fought for it until the very end. *A leukaemia*, the doctor had said, first lesson in the medical language we were shortly to learn. So: more than one type of leukaemia; so: perhaps we had the better type. The scene sketched itself in both our heads as we walked across Archbishop's Park, past the deserted football pitches, and the playground where we'd once watched our children cling to the roundabout. 'Yes, you'll need regular check-ups,' we could imagine a doctor saying, 'but this is really very common.' It didn't seem impossible. In our imaginations, regular check-ups – or whatever this crisis demanded – felt like a concession to what had happened, a down payment to show our fantasy wasn't too childish. That was how we balanced reality with hope, in the hours ahead.

Nicola walked steadily alongside me. I talked to comfort her. We kept step in our instinct to be calm, but around us the clouds were melting, the trees withering. We didn't look at them. More dreadful by far was the fissure that had opened between us, a hairline crack. For nearly thirty years we had done everything together: lived, loved, raised children. Now a summons had come. One of us had been called away. It was in Nicola's blood that the rogue cells were surging and darkly multiplying, even as we walked past the heavy summer trees, laden with leaves, past the gardeners' shed with a mower parked outside it. It was Nicola, not I, who would lie on an operating couch, an hour later, while a young doctor in a blue plastic apron pecked at her spine with a needle, trying to dredge up some of those rogue cells for analysis.

We were scared together; we faced cancer together. But the cancer was poisoning her blood, not mine. It was

Nicola who would die, thirteen months later, with a tube in her throat and her lips weakly fluttering as she tried to smile at me.

'The surgery called ahead,' we told the nurse on reception at A&E.

'Have you been here before, dear?'

The kindliness of the NHS; its dowdy efficiency. The nurse tapped at a keyboard held together with tape. Around us sat the clients of St Thomas's A&E: a Sudanese family in robes, grandfather leaning his hands on a stick, two girls swinging their legs; a drunk slumped across plastic chairs; a burly, bandaged man in a high-vis. Rubber tyres squeaked on the lino. An old man was pushed past on a gurney, naked shoulders as brown as leather and a drip swinging above his head. I watched Nicola's eyes following him, and knew what she was thinking: this was the company she had joined, her new family of the sick. How, in a moment, could so much status be lost? Nicola was a leading figure in the arts. She wasn't a proud or arrogant person – the very opposite. But we saw the world from the modest heights we had scaled together, living among rooftops and terraces, not in luxury but above the city's gutters. Now we were jostling along in the crowd of suffering, coughing, sickening humanity. Blood cells respect no class or salary, thank God. We were just ordinary patients, a sick woman and a frightened husband.

We confirmed our GP's address. Someone got Nicola a wheelchair, though she didn't feel ill, just scared. And we both knew, without saying it, that this was where we needed to be, among other people who faced what we faced. Since we had no entitlement to health, nor should we expect any other special treatment.

'The doctor will be a few minutes.'

The doctor had tousled hair and looked barely older than our son. His natural expression was a friendly grin, although he tried his best to look concerned. They wheeled Nicola into a ward at the back of A&E, half-darkened. They needed white cells from her bone marrow.

I sat hunched on a chair and watched, from a distance, as her torment began. My wife's smooth and lovely body transformed, suddenly, into something for medics to examine and analyse, a broken thing that needed to be fixed. I couldn't see her, just the doctor's back, and the shape made by her legs. The lights were dimmed. I clutched her grey coat on my knees, the coat she had put on that morning in a different world – breakfast snatched, a coat flung on the shoulders. Twenty minutes, they had said. I read anxiety in the hunch of the young doctor's shoulders. He'd already been half an hour. I realised that I needed to cry. I went out along corridors past parked gurneys, out through swing doors into the hospital's labyrinth. In an old marble hall my footsteps echoed oddly behind me, as if their tuning or timing had been subtly changed. Memorial boards listed the dead. The marble heads of doctors stared past me. An old woman in a dressing gown shuffled along on a zimmer frame. I found a glass door opening onto a dark garden. I hadn't realised night had fallen – we must have been in A&E for hours already. A passing cleaner glanced at me, then went back to pushing his mop across the floor. I wasn't sure if I was supposed to be there, but opened the door and went out.

The silhouette of a chapel loomed above me. I was in one of the courtyards between the blocks of old St Thomas's. In front of me was a terrace with the river slipping beyond. The clouds overhead were orange.

I sat down on a bench, barely able to breathe. The noise I made was thin and unnatural. I wasn't good at crying – I wasn't used to it, I'd had so little to cry about. I had cried after my father's stroke, and Nicola had held me in bed, comforting me. I cried again when he died, conventional tears dampening my wife's soft neck. The tears I wept now were ugly and harsh, dredged up from inside me, as painful as bile. I tried to grab hold of what was happening, of what I needed to do. I couldn't. It felt as if time was burning through my fingers, searing them when I tried to slow it. Nicola's illness in Madrid – the bruises on her leg – more than one type of leukaemia. There was no abacus on which to compute this data. She lay inside with a doctor stabbing needles into her bone. Buildings after an earthquake stay crazily upright, stairs climbing to nothing and bathrooms exposed. Our life felt like that – shaken once, viciously, but still standing; insecure.

I looked at the roofs of Parliament, lit up orange. If I were to walk up to the parapet I would see Big Ben, its face hanging in the sky like a second moon. Our children had been born in this hospital. The seventh floor – or was it Room Seven on some other floor? A corner room with big windows staring at Big Ben, so that we could read the time of their birth from its ivory face. The midwife's name was Myrtle. She delivered both of our children, two years apart. With our first, Martha, we had no idea how we would feel as parents. I could remember Nicola coming down to the pool at her parents' house in France, on a summer holiday, holding the plastic pregnancy kit and crying. We had made something together, a living embodiment of love, and as logical in its sequence as our first kiss, or the first time we slept together. Nicola had never quite trusted her body. She was too fat in girlhood, she thought. She was no sportswoman. But in pregnancy she was graceful. Her walk slowed to an unhurried amble. Her face glowed. She gave birth to Martha kneeling, fingers gripping mine as I smoothed her damp hair. Her cry of pain came from somewhere deep and unsophisticated, from the more ancient woman within her polished self. Her chest heaved under the hospital gown. Her shoulders were slick with sweat.

'Well done, Nicola. Give me another push.'

Pain that gave life. 'A girl, a little girl.'

Shrivelled in the midwife's hands, fists clenched, eyes tightly shut. Outside, in a different world, the hands on Big Ben pointed to seven-twenty and people walked past on Westminster Bridge. It was the start of the most wonderful adventure of our lives together. Parenthood slowed and deepened Nicola. We both felt a contentment we had never dreamed possible, in each other and in our lives. It was slower than first love and more deep-rooted, binding us together under the soil. Two years later, Joe was born in the same room at six in the morning. Myrtle drove me home. Our new son kicked in a crib while Nicola tried to sleep – she had been torn. I found her holding him, a few hours later, with a furious love that would have made me jealous if I hadn't shared it myself.

'Was it awful?'

'It was fine.' A reassuring squeeze of my hand.

The doctor looked exhausted. 'We couldn't get a sample, unfortunately. The white cells are packed so tight I couldn't get the needle in. It sometimes happens like that.'

A consultant came. His face was deep-lined and his manner learned. He nodded and smiled as Nicola described symptoms, not listening. He explained, without explaining anything. Nicola sat up against the pillows, bright-eyed, smiling and lucid, her courage fuelled by adrenaline.

'Our son starts his A-levels on Tuesday week,' she said. 'I think I ought to delay treatment until after the exams.'

The consultant shook his head straightaway. His answer was carefully phrased. 'I have to tell you,' he said, 'that you are in a life-threatening situation.'

They put her on a darkened ward, awaiting transport to the blood cancer unit at Guy's. I sat on a chair outside, hoping she'd sleep. The hospital's small dramas went on around us as we waited. Most of the beds were empty, but on one an old man, drunk, lay moaning. The nurses seemed to know him. Little by little the story emerged. He was homeless. He checked into different A&Es each night to get a bed, using a false name.

'You were here last night, Harry.'

He moaned, drunk, or pretending to be. The dimmed light washed over one side of his face, an unshaven cheek. Silence, then a sudden yell, unguarded as a child's.

'It hurts … it hu-urts.'

Outside, in the glaring overhead lights, they loaded Nicola onto an ambulance to drive her to Guy's. The office blocks stood tall around the hospital; the street was quiet. Dead night. Only the bright cavern of the ambulance hollowed out the tarmac darkness, a hole of bright light illuminating oxygen bottles and masks, scuffed lino, a red blanket folded on the gurney. A single whoop on the siren, and we hung in a queue, blocked by the vehicle in front.

Nicola managed a smile. We'd lived in these streets for twenty-eight years; they were home. The year we married, we found a derelict house on Kennington Road. We moved between friends' flats while the builders re-roofed and wired it, cut out rot. We held a decorating party: bowls of pasta and salad in return for paint daubed on skirtings and walls. Five years later we took Martha back there from this same hospital ramp, and it became a quieter place, filled with the chemical smells of washing and nappies. We got a short-legged antique nursing chair from somewhere, and I found Nicola on it at three in the morning, legs sprawled, nose in a book, while the tight bundle of blanket in her lap shifted as Martha suckled. Neither of us could believe the miracle of her body giving life. Our daughter peered at us through the slats of her cot. Her weight in the Moses basket, as I swung it to make her sleep, seemed like the weight of planets orbiting a sun. When Joe was born we had to go into hospital when complications threatened. Nicola had a contraction halfway to the car and leaned against the bus stop, fingers gripping concrete, until it had passed.

Our streets. The driver nosed through them, blue light flashing on the white line ahead, parked cars, closed shops. Inside Nicola's body now, the furious mystery of her approaching death. We didn't know it. Every instinct we had yearned towards hope, but fog had descended, thick as the yellow fog of the streetlights. We knew nothing about leukaemia, or being ill. *You are in a life-threatening situation*. It was hard to understand how we'd travelled so far so quickly. When Nicola felt ill, three weeks before, the doctor had diagnosed a virus, reasonably enough, and prescribed antibiotics. She'd taken them in our hotel bedroom in Madrid, then strode out valiantly to see the Goyas in the Prado. On the way home our flight had been delayed, and we'd texted a photo home, the two of us grinning in the airport. Nicola was already dying, although we didn't know it then, and couldn't see it now; just felt the cold breath of it around us.

Leukaemia.

The entrance to Guy's was cold and empty, awash with fluorescent light. 'We've found a bed,' the doctor said, as if all the beds had been hiding. A ward on an upper floor, hidden within labyrinthine corridors, masked by signs I would only learn later. It took time for the porter to find a nurse.

'We'll just keep you here one night, then move you onto the ward.'

And suddenly we realised this was our new horizon: from now on we would live one day, one night at a time. This was our new perspective. Until six hours before, the months had receded into a tidy future, joys and petty challenges laid out for us like side chapels along the nave of a church. We'd had a weekend planned; I was due to start my new job on Monday; our daughter's exams began on Tuesday, and our son's the week after that. For June we'd booked a holiday in Greece, and in October we'd go to Nicola's parents' house in France. It all seemed so orderly, as if preordained. Suddenly that neat perspective was gone, and all certainty had vanished with it.

I helped Nicola pull off her socks. Her back hurt from the needle earlier. She dropped her clothes on the floor: her skirt, her top, the necklace she'd put on that morning. It felt like watching a prisoner hand in wristwatch and wallet to the guards. She pulled on a blue hospital gown. The sheet was hard and dead, all softness boiled out of it along with the patients' germs. She lay down on her side, tired out.

'I want to stay with her.'

'Of course.'

I pulled up a chair next to the bed. My wife's hip lifted the blanket in front of me. Beyond her an anglepoise lamp stood guard over rows of electrical sockets and the spigot for an oxygen line. Light slatted through the blind. We held hands. Around us, outside the thin pleated curtain that traced our new home, we could hear nurses moving between beds, the squeak of a trolley wheel on the rubber floor, and a bleating of instruments like the chirrup of birds in a marsh. We didn't talk; Nicola had to sleep. And we both needed time, in any case, to find words for what was happening.

I thought of the television news we'd watched the night before, about Syrian refugees arriving on a Greek island. Houses blasted and homes gone, they reached the beach carrying exhausted children and bundles of clothes and valuables, the rescued debris of once-happy lives. In the camps they found homes wherever they could, staking out a gap between two tents, or a few metres of tarmac. One can invent a home anywhere. The eye draws its own boundaries; a scrap of sheet on a clothes line can become the wall of an imagined house.

That was the sort of haven we'd reached now. As the night passed, the wooden arm of my chair started to feel familiar, almost reassuring. I took comfort in a jagged shadow on the curtain. So long as the shadow didn't move, then time stood still; we were alive.

Nicola and I had always been good at making homes. We made our first the first night we slept together, twenty-eight years before. Afterwards we lay rigid, full of joy but horribly uncomfortable on the narrow futon. The room's only window was a rooflight, uncurtained. Lying together we could see the sky over London. Nicola's jeans dangled from the chair; there was a pile of books on the desk, and a scatter of make-up: all the intimacies of another person's life. My work bag lay in one corner, an intruder. Time hung still. One night together, and already we'd built our first home from a room of tousled clothes.

Later Nicola moved in with me. Giving her the keys to my flat in Battersea was the first ritual of our marriage. Then we found the derelict in Kennington; and moved again, seven years later, into another across the road. It was uninhabitable. There were no floorboards in the living room, and an old man had made his home on the ground floor, in the room we would turn into a kitchen. He kept a pet pigeon whose droppings covered the floor. A family with a newborn baby and a cat, we camped in the only finished rooms, up in the attic. For a week we had no kitchen and barbecued in the huge, weed-choked garden, where a mulberry tree threw shade over a patch of rubble, stacks of copper piping, the builders' iron lock-up. I fitted the kitchen the weekend Princess Diana died. The cat, terrified, hid under the floorboards for three days.

Now, sitting behind a curtain in the hospital ward, it was as if our life had returned to its starting point: abandoned clothes, light on the ceiling. Nicola cleared her throat, halfway in or out of sleep. Once, that sound had been new, strange and exciting; now it was as familiar to me as my own breath. The curve of her body was imprinted on my hand. The shape of her lips when she smiled was the sight I knew best in the world. For twenty-eight years it was Nicola who had really been my home.

At dawn I walked home to fetch pyjamas, books and a toothbrush. I leant against the wall in Tabard Alley, the narrow lane between Guy's and Borough High Street, and cried again. I noticed a plaque on the wall: it was the place from where Chaucer's pilgrims had set out on their journey in *The Canterbury Tales*. Out of doors, my crying sounded thin, like the mew of a gull. Taxis sighed past on Borough High Street. It was still half-dark.

I'd meant to walk, but flagged a cab down. The driver could see I didn't want to talk. We drove past the office where I was due to start my new job after the weekend. Craning round, I could see Guy's tower in the rear window. London echoed around me. It wasn't even a full day since Nicola had been diagnosed. When I looked at my hand, it was tremulous and white, without strength. The scrape of my key in the door almost made me cry again. That would be the hardest part of all, after I lost her, coming home from work to an empty house that had once been filled with life and noise. The hall was empty now – Joe was asleep upstairs.

The thought of telling our children filled me with dread. I put on the kettle, showered. Thought of Nicola among strangers, with the blue hospital lights around her and the terror of uncertainty that fills all patients, everywhere: *What is happening to me? What will happen next?* I needed to be with her, but I also needed sleep.

I didn't sleep, of course. The bed was half-empty, the chest of drawers silent and reproachful. Her shirt lay on the chair as if it had been washed up after a storm. A hurricane passing through the house, through our lives, overturning chairs, ripping pictures from walls and returning it to dereliction.

I went into the bathroom and leaned on the cold white china handbasin. Nicola's make-up, her hairbrush, a spongebag lying open to reveal lipstick and eyeliner. Over the next year, our bedroom and bathroom would fill with the strange paraphernalia of sickness: boxes of paracetamol, a thermometer, the scarves she used when her hair went. We tried to treat them as honoured guests. It was part of our quest to make what was happening seem ordinary. At the time, we imagined that would make it easier to bear, so we welcomed the stacks of pills, and the hospital publications – *Eating with Neutropenia* – just as we refused to be scared by the new language that colonised our life of words together: platelets and counts, neutrophils, remission. Like an aeroplane suddenly shifting course in mid-air, its white trail kinked to track a new direction across the sky, we treated illness as no more than a change in direction. We accepted it in our lives, built it into our home like bricklayers mortaring stones into a wall. A survivable cancer, we told ourselves, can be part of being normal. Now I know death is normal too.

I thought of wars, sometimes, in the first few weeks. Young men born in the 1890s found themselves destined for the trenches; born thirty years later, they fought in the Second World War. Neither chose to belong to generations that went to war, but it made no difference. *Why me? Why us?* were never helpful questions. Things happen; people, in the end, are small, and our own sense that we can govern our lives' direction is an illusion borne of fifty years' peace and prosperity.

It seemed no more helpful, now, to ask *Why us?* Neither of us ever felt angry about cancer. At Nicola's memorial celebration, in London's Roundhouse, our friend Marcus wrote a beautiful panegyric of a woman whose colleagues and friends in the arts loved her as much as her family did. We talked beforehand and agreed we didn't want anger in the room. Cancer was just something that happened to us.

When I heard Joe going down to the kitchen, I got up and followed him. I don't remember exactly what I said. He was eighteen, then, with A-levels looming in front of him. I didn't hold off from using the C-word, *Cancer.* His face stayed calm. I knew I could rely on Joe's strength – I've relied on it ever since.

We'd had two years with our son after Martha went to university. He'd used them to mature, ducking out from under an older sister's shadow, and growing closer to us. In those two years Joe had found a new assurance, something like Nicola's comfort in her own skin. He and Nicola had always been close; she was Joe's ally when we were together as a family. While Martha and I tended to be frenetic and driven, Nicola and Joe shared an inner calm. Now, Joe took the news of her illness in his stride. I said there were different types of leukaemia. He nodded and asked a few questions, not many.

Like his mother, he had the natural grace to know when not to ask too much. Besides, he had a younger sibling's instinct to take things back to his room, where he could contemplate them without interference. He would process this news in his own way, I knew.

I texted Nicola: *Just told Joe. He's coming with me at 12.*

The nurse had said not to return before then. Doctors would need to visit, tests to be taken.

I texted: *Told him we were going to withhold scary words from M, and he's OK with that.*

Martha faced exams the next day. Neither of us wanted to talk of *cancer* and *leukaemia* over the phone. Besides, we had no firm news; we hadn't yet seen the consultants. Maybe it was nothing, like the friend at work who lived with leukaemia under control. The consultant in A&E had told us what they thought it was: Acute Myeloid Leukaemia (AML). It was the first time we'd heard the name. We still didn't know what it meant.

I told Martha something was wrong but they weren't sure what. There was nothing to worry about.

'They're keeping her in,' I said over the phone.

'Why?' My daughter's voice sounded very small and far away. I wanted to hug her, as if she was still a little girl.

'They're doing tests,' I added, not answering the question. 'To see what's going on.'

Afterwards, Martha told me she knew straightaway it was something like cancer. Or at least some part of her knew –

but she allowed herself to believe our fiction. I think that was the last time she let herself be treated as a child.

It was different a year later, when Nicola was sinking in intensive care. Martha, Joe and I went into the consultant's office together. Our children didn't want to be shielded from what was happening; they were part of it. We held hands as the consultant told us there was nothing more they could do. He was Italian, a burly man trying not to cry. I could feel Martha and Joe on either side of me as I nodded, asked for some details, thanked him for explaining how she was. Joe asked how long she might have. Martha squeezed my hand.

The consultant said, 'We can leave her as she is and she will sink slowly. Perhaps it will take a few hours. Or we can switch off the machines and let her go now.'

'There's no doubt?' I asked. My voice didn't sound like my usual voice.

He said, 'No.'

I looked at Martha, who nodded, then at Joe, who did the same. Then I said firmly, 'We want to let her go now.'

Both their childhoods were over by then. A month after Nicola's death we went away to travel together, bound in grief, buoyed by her strength.

2

On the first morning of Nicola's illness I texted, *How r u feeling?* Her response came cheerfully back: *Feeling fine!* By the time Joe and I reached Guy's they'd moved her to a new ward: Samaritan.

Over the next year, Samaritan Ward would become a part of our lives. It was one of the kindest places I've ever known. Kind but shabby; the staff told us it was due for refurbishment. The vinyl flooring was cracked and the paint faded; notices blu-tacked untidily to the walls of its long, dim corridor warned of infection, untested appliances, and the hot water in the tea caddy. A board of staff mugshots surrounded 'Nurse of the Month' in a frame. To either side, doors led to single rooms. At the centre of the ward stood a desk where medical staff tapped at ageing laptops with anglepoise lamps bowed solicitously above them. Open wards, barely wider than corridors, stretched out in two directions. At mealtimes dinner ladies rolled trolleys slowly from bed to bed, wafting behind them a thick smell of hospital food.

On that Saturday morning I found Nicola sitting up in bed on the open ward. I off-loaded pyjamas and clean knickers, a stack of books, a cotton bag containing play-texts she was judging for a competition. She grinned and kissed me.

'I don't feel ill at all,' she complained.

Doctors had been and more were coming. They'd move her into her own room, they said, as soon as the treatment started – they'd need to guard her against infection. That was our first lesson in cancer treatment: chemotherapy reduces immunity. The treatment could be almost as dangerous as the disease. *Neutropenia*, induced by the chemo, was the flattening of the body's immune system. A city without walls, the body's streets become prey to the infections that lurk in cellars and alleyways, that crawl up from gutters, that live among us, killers, unseen. That would one day kill Nicola, who sat on her bed listing books I should bring. In the first days of her illness, she still had energy, and a fierce will to make illness treat her with respect. She would manage this, she decided, the way she managed the shows she produced: cheerfully and without giving in to stress. So she wanted comfort-reading; she wanted pictures to look at; she wanted her tapestry. I took notes: the hand cream in the bathroom; the grey top without sleeves.

We met the consultant that evening, a lean man ten years older than us. He wrapped his hands around his legs and spoke breezily, comfortingly, of tried-and-tested courses of treatment. His tone was bracing and faintly gung-ho. 'We can deal with this' was one phrase we seized on, the lifting of a death sentence neither of us had acknowledged to be there.

The treatment would start straightaway, Dr Clay said. As he unwrapped himself and stood up, he added, 'We'll give those cancer cells something to think about.'

'It's going to be all right,' we repeated to each other. It wasn't mere bravado, or forlorn hope. We were each letting the other know we weren't giving in to despair, or panic, or gloom. Hope would be our *Marseillaise*, stirring us to rise each morning, strengthening us through good tests and bad, through setbacks and disappointments. We never knew Nicola was dying. I have friends who've nursed partners through terminal illness where they knew the end was coming. It was worse for them, I think. We never knew there was an end until the very last days of Nicola's life.

And with cancer and the risk of death would grow the deepest love we had ever known. Welded to each other like lovers on a hillside, we had eyes, lips, only for one another. Cancer was a storm raging furiously around us. Love was the hut in which we found shelter. Shabby enough, but on a bed laid in one corner we had never held each other so tightly nor felt so intensely each other's warmth. I can't feel anger, writing this six months after Nicola died. Much later, I spoke to a friend who had nursed his wife through terminal illness. He said, 'Caring for someone you love when they're dying is the biggest thing you can give them.' There seems no more point regretting illness than regretting a war or an earthquake. We loved each other perfectly while Nicola was alive.

On Sunday morning I pulled knickers from her drawer and worked out what she meant by the grey top without sleeves. I loaded the washing machine and sent her a Snapchat of heaped pyjamas to boast how much I'd done. After twenty-eight years and two children, we thought our intimacy was complete. Sickness deepened it.

Back at Guy's I found Nicola had been moved into a room with a view of St Paul's Cathedral. The room was small and square, too small for the fridge, which stood in one corner getting in everyone's way, or the bedside table, which wandered to and fro on rebellious castors. In the centre was a bed, the room's masterpiece, an engineering miracle able to roll, incline or hoist patients to any conceivable angle or position. It must have been designed for massive American private hospitals. Squeezed into Nicola's tiny cell, its headboard struck the anglepoise when she sat up, and its foot caught on the fridge when the nurses tried to lift her. Visitors sitting on the chair hit the control pad with their knees, raising her head uncontrollably, or rolling her from left to right while she tried frantically to reach the remote.

I stacked books on the window shelf. Peering down, we could see the roofs of cars, and doctors crossing the courtyard. It was the long view that captivated her, though. St Paul's sailed majestically along the horizon, a liner heading for a foreign port. Later, I brought in pencil and paper and Nicola sketched it inexpertly. Each morning she sent me the same photograph of it, lit afresh by the sunrise, while at night I received blurry Snapchats of the illuminated dome, like an amateur astronomer's pictures of the rings of Saturn.

That Sunday morning we looked out of the window and counted the spires of Wren churches, mementoes of an older, sweeter London disappearing under tumorous office blocks. We could see cars, pedestrians, the corner of a street. A life from which we had suddenly withdrawn continued beyond glass, inaudible. Nicola had cried, she admitted, while I'd been away, collecting her things. She introduced me to the nurse who had comforted her, an older woman, a Londoner with a cackling laugh.

'We had a good old weep,' she said, 'didn't we, gel?'

No one had ever called Nicola 'gel' before. We tried to laugh about that, along with the absurdities of the hospital timetable, the television which unaccountably switched itself on and off, and the notice on the fridge which warned against fruit.

'But now I feel fine,' Nicola insisted. 'Really. Fine.'

I had brought in volumes of paintings and drawings. We pinned photographs to the noticeboard. On the wall above the bed hung a picture of a sunset. I filled the fridge with lemonade and Coke bought in the shop downstairs. Our radio perched on her shelf, missing home. We spent Sunday afternoon playing cards. It was only two days since Nicola's ordeal had begun, and already we were slipping into the routines of illness.

On Monday I started my new job.

I sought out one of the partners in the architectural practice I was joining, and told him, standing on the staircase, that my wife had just been diagnosed with cancer. People, strangers, shuffled past us on their way to their desks. His face creased with concern. From the outset, my new practice couldn't have been more supportive. It was never going to feel normal, though, to sit in the training room being inducted in the email system and the office diary; or to email clients; or sketch over the concert hall I was working on in Edinburgh. *Boy, am I inducted*, I texted Nicola late Monday morning. She responded, *Ha ha starting to feel the same way*. Architectural models crowded the shelves. The office banter eddied around a new face. I didn't tell anyone else that my wife was ill.

Monday lunchtime, I walked up Southwark Street to the hospital, crossed the bustling reception full of relatives and hurrying doctors, stopped for the lift that went up to the cancer ward. While I waited for someone to answer the bell, I peered through the window at Samaritan, the strange island to which Nicola had been banished. A tea trolley stood askew between two open doors. A patient in a pink gown, bald, shuffled painfully along on a zimmer frame. The world of architecture seemed impossibly far away. It was like peering in on someone else's dream.

I found Nicola sitting cross-legged on her bed, stitching at a tapestry cushion cover with the newspaper spread around her. Her mother had been to see her, she told me. All weekend she'd been dreading it, but now she seemed relieved.

Nicola was her mother's only child, though her father had children from a previous marriage. She and Anne, her mother, were close. It wasn't so much that they were alike in character – Nicola had more of her father's calm than her mother's boundless energy and willpower. But Anne and Peter had, between them, created the world in which Nicola grew up, and we both shared its values.

I first met them when I was nineteen and Nicola, a new friend, asked me round one evening. I'd never come across grown-ups who were so interested in others. Peter handed me the strongest gin and tonic I'd ever drunk. Anne came out of the kitchen, from which emerged fragrant smells of something cooking in wine, and introduced me to a group of people of all ages – some friends of Nicola's and others of theirs. Modern art hung on the walls. A huge vase of flowers nodded white blooms above an antique sideboard. One thing became clear straightaway: that I was expected to talk. Dullness, laziness, self-indulgence, lack of humour – those were the great crimes around Anne's and Peter's dinner table. Later, I understood them better: they hated people who were false, dishonest or pretentious; they treasured kindness and good judgement. What was immediately apparent, though, was the value they placed on talking. It might have seemed contrived to our children's generation. It wasn't, in Clarendon Road, as glasses were filled and Anne brought course after course of delicious food from the tiny kitchen no one else was allowed to enter. Conversation was the common ground on which different people met; the place ideas could be turned over. It was food for the mind. The talk slipped easily into laughter – pretentiousness was as unwelcome as ignorance – but silence was never allowed to fall. That was the world in which Nicola had grown up, a world in which words were valued and beauty cherished, where ideas were welcome, rather than intimidating. She'd absorbed it without ever realising it, and friends like myself learned it in turn.

On that first hospital visit, Nicola told me, her mother had brought books and food. She had talked about the practicalities of letting people know, worried about money, then stopped so as not to be seen worrying. I knew she would have taken in everything – the crow's feet of tiredness by her daughter's eyes, the determination in her voice. I imagine she wept outside.

Throughout Nicola's illness, Anne's role was harder than mine. I, at least, could be by Nicola's side, helping her through each day. Anne wouldn't let herself intrude. When Nicola was in intensive care, a year later, I used to visit before work, then call Anne from the hospital steps.

She tried to hold herself back from cross-examining me, but failed, of course.

'So she's better?'

'She's the same. She's not worse, and that's good news.'

'But she'll get better?'

'The doctors hope so, but it's going to be slow, Anne.'

'So at least she's steady?'

Yearning for good news like water in a desert, for good news that I couldn't always supply, she had to watch from aside as her only daughter sickened and died.

On that first visit Anne had brought grapes, even though grapes were not allowed, banned flowers, and piles of books that would have daunted even someone in perfect health.

'She was great,' Nicola said. 'She's being really strong. Now I'm exhausted.'

Nothing more tiring than worrying about people who are worrying about you. That evening, when I visited again after work, we sent an email to our friends:

This is to let you all know that, although everything's going to be fine, Nicola's been diagnosed with a strain of leukaemia, and is in Guy's at the moment, having treatment. Everyone is being fantastically positive, not least Nicola herself. The doctors are relaxed. There are many forms of leukaemia, and they're confident of sorting this out. But it will be a rough six months, in and out of hospital.

Sorry not to have called you individually. Very selfishly, we'd rather you managed any shock by yourselves, and then came out being as positive as the four of us all are. In due course Nicola, who's fine at the moment, would love calls, texts and emails to help fight the boredom. But don't be offended if she doesn't pick up.

Much love to you all. Nicola really wants me to stress that she's okay – and indeed she's looking very cheerful in bed at the moment, with piles of books and a view of St Paul's.

That night Nicola texted: *Alison Balsom, sudoku, patience, and quite a large supper.* I'd given her Alison Balsom's trumpet recordings of Bach for Christmas. At home, tired from my first day at work, I cooked Joe spare ribs, and we drank beer and watched *True Grit.* Nicola texted, *No reaction at all so far.*

The chemo had started straightaway. They'd put in a 'Hickman line'. I'd seen it when I visited on Monday evening: three white plastic tubes trailing from Nicola's chest. The nurses could take blood from them, and pump in chemicals to kill the cancerous cells that were multiplying in her bloodstream and bone marrow. Somehow the Hickman line had brought it home to us that we were in for a long haul.

'Four courses of treatment,' the doctor in A&E had said. 'Normally. You need to allow six months.'

Six months. It sounded forever, at the time. We lived in a world where things happened fast.

We asked Dr Clay about it when he visited that evening. Could it really take six months?

'Cancer's hard to predict,' he shrugged. 'Everyone's different.'

Neither of us could get used to losing control over our own lives, but his message was not to count the days. We had to let cancer tug us away from the shore of everyday life. Drifting on a raft, without rudder or oars, all we could do was revolve on the current and watch the shore recede. It was a difficult lesson for two people who liked to be in control, but in the days that followed we realised we had no choice. Overnight we slowed from endless activity, from days of work and evenings seeing friends or going to shows, to the slow monotony of illness.

I cancelled our holiday in Greece. I emailed everyone to postpone our anniversary party, without mentioning cancer. Nicola's only rhythm was the rise of the sun on St Paul's dome each morning, and the halting sequence of doctors' visits. Our days were punctuated by things beyond our control: unpredictable tests, results that came slowly and incomprehensibly. Fog fell. We found ourselves cocooned in it together.

In our new life, everything repeated itself: the hospital door's slow revolve, the wait for the lift, the ringing of the bell outside Samaritan.

I learned the ritual of protective clothing needed to protect Nicola from infection as chemotherapy dismantled her immune system. Outside her room, each day, I washed my hands, tore a blue plastic apron from the roll above the sink, and drew rubber gloves onto my fingers. Only then could I tap on the door and go in. Doctors visited at unforeseeable moments. We rarely understood what they told us – blood cancer is complex medicine. We didn't know what AML was, or how blood counts worked. We found ourselves adrift and out of our depth on this unknown ocean, cancer, with no chart to guide us. Nothing was quite clear. One doctor mentioned four weeks' recovery time from chemotherapy, another said five. One mentioned more tests to be done; another seemed to think they knew enough. We scanned each phrase for clues, like priests trying to read the future in clouds.

Of course, we could have gone online to research, but shared an instinct not to. We wanted neither tales of medical disaster nor miracle cures, and dreaded the cocky self-assurance of internet oracles. Instead we chose to trust our consultants, and the tired, cheerful nurses who tapped on Nicola's door, every hour, to take her 'obvs' – her 'observations', blood pressure and temperature – or bent over her Hickman line to squeeze in the deadly chemicals that would save her. It was their professionalism and quiet care we needed, not the shrill clamour of the internet.

Trust was what we needed: trust in our family, in each other, in the people caring for Nicola. Trust was Nicola's instinct – it was how she worked in her theatre life. She didn't bully people, measure them, set targets for them; she trusted them, and she would trust her doctors too. In the thirteen months of her illness, nothing made us regret that choice.

There were no certainties, though. Dr Clay had said Nicola's cancer was usually curable. It was still cancer. Samaritan Ward was full of the very sick. Children lost in a forest, we had entered death's realm, and we knew it. A week in, and feeling reassured by the prognosis, we cautiously allowed ourselves to look ahead. The cloud lifted just far enough for us to talk of 'next weekend', and 'after this treatment'. It made everything worse. For one horrible weekend we worried and couldn't talk. Nicola cried for the second time since she was diagnosed.

That was when we realised we didn't want to look into the future. We were no longer welcome there: the future was a garden from which we'd been cast out. We couldn't assume a cure – that would be tempting fate. But the alternative, of accepting Nicola might die, was something neither of us could face. A few days later she developed a slight infection. Suddenly she was in danger again – and with relief we fell back into the timeless dreamworld of the sick.

Days blurred. Sometimes the doctors let Nicola out for lunch, wearing a mask. We met in the old garden courtyard of Guy's. Deep within a part of London we thought we knew well, it was a little haven of peace. Nurses sat on the grass eating sandwiches; poppies fringed the lawn; everyone talked quietly. The stone arch at one end had come from old London Bridge. The modern city, roaring around us, seemed a hundred miles away. We found ourselves in the eighteenth century, in Wren's London or Hogarth's. Slowly we walked along the cloister, prisoners enjoying the sun. We developed prisoners' routines, convicts' habits. There was an Italian café we went to on Saturdays, where they served lasagne and plates of tired salad, Coke from the fridge. We walked to the far end of Memorial Park, turned at the gate and walked back again.

Martha came to visit from Cambridge; Joe skyped between revision periods. His exams went past, one by one. At home, as the summer warmed up, friends took over our garden, trying to keep things in order for when Nicola was released. They pruned, fed pots, sprayed chemicals. I emailed Nicola photographs of flowers as they came out, one by one – Iris,

Potentilla, Solomon's Seal — snapshots of the summer she was missing. It seemed odd being out there without her; the garden was Nicola's realm. I stared at plants whose names I didn't know, at thickets of swelling greenery that might or might not be prunable. Nicola watched an old DVD of *Bleak House*, and texted me before she went to sleep. *Sleep well loveliest most wonderful one*, she wrote. I texted back, *Honey sleep well I love you so much xxxxxx*.

There might have been something idyllic about this drifting, timeless existence; but the thought of cancer never left us. One day, out on the ward, an old woman died. The nurses were quiet when they took Nicola's obvs. They were upset. We'd imagined that somehow they became hardened to death, working on a cancer ward. But for a day or so you could see grief in their faces, as if death's presence in the ward had suddenly become too palpable, like the reek of a fox on a lawn.

Gradually, almost imperceptibly, the weeks went past. Nicola counted down her twice-daily chemo. At last she texted, *Done*. Her first round of chemotherapy was over.

The treatment was over, but in some ways the hardest part was still to come. Nicola's neutrophils — the measure of her immune system — would fall as she descended into neutropenia, then rise again to return her to safety. But for as long as she was neutropenic, she was vulnerable to infection.

We waited impatiently for the results of her daily blood samples. As her 'platelet' counts dropped, she needed transfusions. The platelets were yellow and vaguely repulsive, sagging in blisters from the hooks alongside her bed. We soon got used to them. After four weeks, treatment had become ordinary – Nicola had become a patient. She knew the names of the pills in her chest of drawers and what they were for. She had learned how the hospital worked; what she could trust and what could go wrong. Discreetly, she checked whether new platelets had been ordered, whether results had returned. She was a good patient. The sweet personality that made her so skilful a producer had her gossiping with cleaners, chatting with matrons. She was delighted when a masseur turned up at her door, sent by Dimbleby Cancer Care, to give her a foot massage.

The day Nicola's counts started rising, we celebrated. It seemed like proof that treatment was predictable after all; that AML was curable; that Nicola was no different from other patients who had left Samaritan, cured, to resume their normal lives. And 'normal' was what we both yearned for. We wanted to wake up in the morning lying next to each other. I wanted to hear the sound of my wife brushing her teeth; the rhythm of light switch and tap so regular, so unchanging that I had never stopped to record it. We wanted to have breakfast in the garden at weekends, or on weekdays, rushing for work. We wanted to have lunch with

Nicola's parents, to go to exhibitions, meet friends at plays. We didn't yearn for anything special. It was the unrecorded minutiae of life that we missed, those actions that you remark no more than you exert the muscles that pump your heart. We wanted the miracle of ordinary health, of breath steadily flowing and our bodies moving easily to pull on socks, brush hair, send an email. We wanted the weariness of watching news at the end of the day, and the pile of washing-up in the sink after dinner. Gradually, in our years together, our habits had formed around us. We wanted them back. Most of all, we wanted to make plans, to choose Christmas presents, to fantasise about holidays we might never take. We wanted to put clothes away, trusting we would get them out again on another occasion; to talk of 'next summer' or 'next year' with the certainty that in time it would come around. We wanted to worry about others, not ourselves. We wanted the sky to unknot, and the earth to stop shaking.

When Nicola came home she was weak as a child. She sat in one corner of the sofa, smaller than she'd been the morning she left for work, six weeks before. Her eyes travelled over the kitchen, the piano and television, delighted to be back.

We'd been delayed leaving the hospital. Nicola had been packed by eight and ready to go, but her drugs weren't prepared. NHS wheels ground slowly. Forms had to be filled in. The dispensary was somewhere else in the vast building. The morning's blood tests had to be logged.

One result, a few days before, had depressed us. Diminished by four hard doses of chemo, Acute Myeloid Leukaemia will normally retreat into remission. Nicola had a blood marker that suggested hers was likely to recur. Not only would she need three more hits of chemo, but a bone marrow transplant, at the end of treatment, to ensure all remained well. We didn't know, then, what a transplant meant. It was the extra time involved that seemed unbearable. Six months had already been lost. The transplant would add another three months, perhaps more – she would probably be off for a year in all.

Dr Clay sounded vague about it. 'I'm not a transplanter,' he said. 'They do the transplants at King's. You'll meet Dr Anand – she knows all about them.'

For a day Nicola had been depressed, but she bounced back with her usual resilience.

Feeling much more cheery, she texted the same evening. *My keyworker nurse confirmed no change to the view this will be cured. Just a more hardcore type of treatment.*

I had scrubbed the house clean for her return. Neutropenic, Nicola would be prey to the bugs and bacteria all around her, so I scrubbed basins and disinfected toilets, rubbed the shine off the kitchen worktop, wiped down light switches, door handles, the knob of the kettle. It felt like I was revisiting all the habits of our life: our hands gliding up the banister to bed, switching off lights, closing doors. The thoughtless ritual of watching television: I ran a wipe over the controls, cleaning the buttons we would press to switch on news or lock in the DVD for our Sunday-evening ritual of pizza and a movie. I wiped down the knobs of her chest of drawers, effacing the mark of however many mornings when she had hastily grabbed knickers or tights, rubbing away the palimpsest of fingermarks that had accumulated invisibly in the house where we had been so happy for nineteen years.

Nicola had clutched her bag on her lap as I drove her home. The short walk from the car had tired her. Now she sat gingerly in one corner of the sofa, a stranger suddenly, whose world, like her clothes, seemed too big for her. She wore a yellow headscarf.

I took a photograph to send to our friends.

A very quick update to let you know that Nicola is back home after the first slug of chemo. Here's a photo. Back in Guy's the week after next, so keep the emails & thoughts coming.

We had two weeks together before the next treatment began. Nicola went to bed early. Pill boxes crowded the table where she kept her books. For some reason I had developed a sore throat. I slept in the basement, taking no chances with infection. From downstairs, forlorn, I texted her good night, as I had when she was in hospital. When my throat recovered, and I could hug her again, I could feel the knobs of her spine like crests of rock breaking through sand. During the day, while I worked, Nicola stitched away at her tapestry, or rested. She took her temperature every few hours, as she'd been instructed. It was early July. Out in the garden, the acanthus was unfurling; oriental poppies shed blowsy petals on the lawn.

Slowly, Nicola's neutrophil counts – the sign of her immune system bouncing back – began to rise. When they reached 1.5 she would officially be out of neutropenia and able to see people again. We celebrated by having friends round to dinner. We'd planned a weekend away – our treat to make up for the summer's lost vacations – but Nicola felt nervous. The fear of infection stalked us. What if something blew up while we were out of London? Normally so confident, Nicola felt brittle. The world seemed dangerous. She didn't want to be too far from the hospital. Samaritan, with its threadbare rhythms and tired faces, now had a familiarity she missed. She missed feeling safe. She missed being cured.

We settled on a day trip to Kent and one night away. I drove us to Penshurst Place, where we'd gone with the children, in the days before we had a garden, to watch them roll across green lawns surrounded by high yew hedges. It was Nicola's favourite type of English garden. As we drove in, wheels trailing plumes of dust from the gravel, roses nodded against a faded brick wall, too high to see over, that ran along one side of the park. Her grandparents had lived in Gloucestershire, in an old stone house with a lawn. Educated at the Lycée, fluent in French, well-travelled, a Londoner to her core, Nicola nevertheless felt the pull of gables and mullioned windows, their Englishness, their familiarity. She had studied the Tudors when she read history at Oxford. We used to play a game of which portraitist we'd pick for each of our friends. For herself she wanted Holbein. Her parents loved old Tudor portraits. One hung in their house, an old woman, thin-lipped, straight-backed, standing on a rush mat and leaning on a cane. At Penshurst we sprawled on the grass. Nicola took a photograph of me. When I look at it now I can see how stressed I was. We wandered through the garden and remembered our children running along the path past the herbaceous border. There was a pub in the village where you could buy food.

From Penshurst we drove west towards the hotel Nicola had booked. The aeroplanes overhead came lower and lower until we found it, eventually, by the perimeter of Gatwick Airport. It didn't matter. The courtyard we drove into was surrounded by thick bushes; the room we were shown had a deep, soft, comfortable bed; and beyond the house, a lawn stretched past shrubs to a quiet pond shaded by willows.

A few times, before we had children, we'd gone away for weekend breaks, but rarely since. In this luxurious place it felt as if we had borrowed other people's lives. The guests were all couples, prosperous, middle-aged. For them a weekend away was nothing special – they would take other weekends, other holidays. And perhaps it was then we realised how much cancer was changing us. Alone among the hotel guests, we had no future we could count on. Tonight was the only time in which we could live: the cool gin and tonics on a tray; the scent of the lawn; the pattern of Nicola's shawl. We had the hope – a real hope – there would be other evenings like this, perhaps many of them. But there was no longer any flow or expanse to the space we lived in. We inhabited it one room at a time, like children straying through a house abandoned by grown-ups, opening cupboards, peering down stairwells.

We sat on a bench together in the garden hemmed in by trees. We didn't envy the other couples. Their powerful cars lined the gravel outside, ready to hurry away. They had money but no time, had time but didn't know its value. They didn't even know how healthy they were. The wine they sipped tasted only of wine; the dishes the waiter unveiled with a florid incantation of ingredients were mere platefuls of food. Perhaps, when they were old, they would try to recall this hotel, and wouldn't even remember the terrace outside with brass-shod chairs, or the shy waitress with red hair, or the ducks swimming on the pond. We, by contrast, would never forget them.

We sat alone in the dining room, marked out by Nicola's headscarf, cancer's uniform. We were marked out from all of them. We had no future, but the present had never seemed so real, or so ancient. We had each other; we were alive. Instead of in a luxurious hotel, we might have been anywhere – on a sea shore, or a bare mountain ledge. The waiter brought our food. It tasted so strong it was almost unbearable. The courgettes were fragrant with life, the meat dark with blood. Nicola pushed her wine glass away: two sips had gone to her head. After dinner we sat out beneath stars that bowed down under their own weight until they hovered just above the grass, and the night, heavy with the scent of flowers, poured sluggishly about us, like a stream flowing through weeds. An aeroplane lowered above us, yearning for the earth.

We drove home next morning, not stopping on the way.

The blood cancer clinic was held on Mondays, early. They took Nicola straight in to start her second round of chemo. She texted me the latest good news: *Bone marrow in remission! I'll call soon.*

'Call soon'. Today the phone lies dead in my pocket. I listen to old messages, sometimes, to hear Nicola's voice. Her words whisper in my ear when I wake up. It seems extraordinary, now she is gone, that the world keeps turning at all. I don't know how the sun can be troubled to rise and set; and yet light stretches along the horizon, each morning, summoning trees and flowers to the weary requirements of another day. I shave, wash, cook. I can feel myself dropping through a void, like a body falling from a tower, or a man in space. Sucked from the capsule in which we lived, Nicola and I hurtle away from one another, lives dwindling to points of light, then darkness.

I woke up last night and when I tried to remember Nicola's face I could recall only the line of her hair, coiling from lock to lock along the side of her sleeping cheek. Which is why I am writing this: to fix words on the page, to close them in darkness before the ink can fade.

3

Our children were partying, that summer. Martha sent photos
of Cambridge balls. She hated the dressing up and formality,
she told us on the phone, but photos showed her radiant. Joe
joined a party on the Thames, texting Nicola as they drifted
past Guy's, with music blaring and lights shining on the oily
surface of the river. Nicola was back in for her second course
of treatment. We watched the summer from her window.
When the hot weather began in earnest, the roof terraces
below us filled up with office parties, sunshades, people
drinking Pimm's and cold beer: tiny, distant figures going
through routines that had once belonged to us. She sketched
St Paul's. Back in Guy's garden, we ate sandwiches perched
on the wall next to beds of poppies. We walked around the
hospital, waiting for her counts to fall again.

There was a chapel in the outer courtyard. Neither of us
had ever been religious, but we both liked visiting churches.
Inside was a lofty eighteenth-century room whose floor and
wooden gallery smelled of wax. Tall windows cast a limpid,

clear light across the rows of pews. Had either of us needed faith, it would have been of this sort: rational, suffused with light.

There was a church we often visited in Suffolk, on the River Deben, that had become one of our favourite places. Its round tower was said to have been used as a lookout against Vikings. Inside were box pews and a high pulpit. The altar was a simple table, and the glass in the windows so old you could see nothing through them; they just admitted light, bathing the worn stone floor, the whitewashed walls that bloomed mould, and the single bellrope looped up in one corner of the tower. There were no statues or saints. Outside, unseen, were the endless sky, and the sea's horizon. The air drifting in through the door smelled of nettles and salt.

We went there on our boat. We'd started sailing when Martha was six and Joe four. I'd grown up with the sea. My father's family had been in the Navy, and my childhood was full of sea stories. As a child I sailed on the Norfolk Broads, and later, out into the North Sea. After my father had a stroke, my mother used to drive him to Shotley Point, so he could look at the sea. The last time I saw him, lying in the hospital at Ipswich, I held his hand and described us sailing down the river, as if I were telling him a story. He couldn't answer, but after a moment he turned his head towards me and tried to smile.

When Martha was six and Joe four, we bought an old boat, *Kismet*, and a larger, even shabbier one, *Zylippe*, when their legs grew too long for its bunks. We sailed to Holland. Halfway across the North Sea, lights shone all around us: stars; the shipping lanes marked out by navigation lights; the dim green glow on our instruments. Black waves lifted and fell about us, unseen. While Martha and I kept watch, Nicola and Joe slept below, wrapped in orange blankets. Everything I cared for and loved was held in that tiny boat rocking on the vast sea, as in a cupped hand. I think it was the happiest moment of my life.

We sailed to be alone together; to make the world shrink; to shut out its din and see further. On our boat there was no telephone or email. We had nothing but each other, books, a basket of food. Sails could take us anywhere; we were cocooned.

Cancer was the same, our cocoon. Or maybe cancer was the dark sea around us.

Nicola went back into Samaritan for her second round of chemo on 13 July. *Call when you can*, she texted. *Am doctor'd, prodded, obsv'd and had a shower.*

The doctors started chemo the same day. This visit shouldn't be so long, they said. They would allow Nicola home when the chemo was done, and we could manage the recovery by ourselves. She had no sign of cancer, the consultant told us; things were going well. The battle now was to make sure leukaemia never came back.

That conflict was waged inside Nicola's body, in her blood: a foreign war, known only through the news reports that arrived on the registrar's laptop. As the drugs took hold again she combed out wisps of hair. The flesh shrank back around the bones of her face and her trousers hung slack about her hips. The hospital food was inedible, she said. Her fingers, stitching away at her tapestry, seemed longer than before; her wedding and engagement rings twisted easily over the joint. When I pressed my cheek against her forehead, at night, I could smell chemicals.

By now, Samaritan Ward had become a second home, a place where we felt at ease. It wasn't faultless, of course. Sometimes prescriptions went astray. Coming to visit, I could find myself stranded outside the locked door for ten minutes – the entryphone was always out of order. But Samaritan was its own strange, kind, shabby universe, and we wouldn't have wanted to be anywhere else. Its people made it special, despite the scuffed lino and the appalling food; despite the broken alarm bleating endlessly along the corridor. At mealtimes, old women pushed trolleys from door to door, talking in the same sweet, soft Jamaican we heard on the bus to Brixton. Many of the nurses were Filipino. We glimpsed how tough their lives were. Most lived far away and the shifts were punishing. It was easy to picture the long bus journeys home to children in crowded flats. On the ward, though, the nurses seemed endlessly happy. They worked without pause, and their commitment was awe-inspiring. One day, the matron discovered that Nicola's nurse didn't know how to give a certain kind of injection so she demonstrated on her own arm and found all the nurses later, in the staff room, practising on themselves.

Many of the nurses became friends. They liked being assigned to Nicola. She talked about their families, gossiped, remembered to thank them for the cleaning, and the drugs and the endless rounds of 'obvs'. Junior doctors lingered awkwardly at the door, hugging sheaves of notes. Nicola's friendliness wasn't polish or empty charm; she had been brought up to care more for people than anything else. She was always more acute about people than me – she saw their faults – but also more forgiving. She expected perfection in no one, found virtues in most. The NHS, that great expression of human kindliness, ground massively around us. We were in awe of it: that it could heal populations and yet cherish individuals, as it cared for her. Next door, cranes revolved over the building site for a new clinic. We told ourselves again and again how lucky we were to be ill at the heart of London, in one of the world's greatest centres for cancer research.

Around us, patients came and went. Old men lay in side rooms, biding time. Newcomers sat up on their beds, eyes shocked and visitors tearful, clutching their hands. We recognised the look on their faces – we'd experienced the same sudden overturning of our own world, seven weeks before. Nicola joked that she felt like an old prisoner when new convicts are brought in.

Sitting dressed on her bed, Nicola emailed friends. We were lucky in our friends. We'd known from the start we could rely on them. Like circus artists trusting the strength of the wires that support them, the safety of the net, we'd been able to let go and fall softly into their arms. They sent books, music, suggestions for television shows. Piles of detective stories built up by Nicola's bed. In the evening she sent me a photo of City lights, taken from her bedroom window. They looked like the lights of ships, floating on a vast black sea.

Our friend Nettie was over from America with her daughters. I cooked a barbecue for her birthday and showed photos to Nicola. We slipped back into the routines of hospital.

At weekends the ward was quiet. The entrance lobby would be deserted when I arrived on Saturday morning, the lifts empty and the corridors pleasantly silent. It felt like entering a kind of haven. We had no parties to go to, no shopping to do, or plays to attend. I would stop at the dingy supermarket for a paper. Sitting in Nicola's visitor chair, unhurried, I would read aloud theatre reviews and foreign news. They sounded like reports from an exotic continent. We did the crossword together. We talked, often about the same things, picking endlessly over Joe's A-levels, or how our children were coping with Nicola's illness. The banalities of a husband's and wife's life together were suddenly precious, now they were under threat, pebbles revealed as gems. Each conversation had a dreadful weight. When I called each morning to ask how Nicola had slept, the answer mattered; it wasn't just a routine question. To fill a bag with socks or shirts was a gift to her more heartfelt than any jewellery or perfume.

On weekdays I visited Nicola each lunchtime. Hurrying from the office, I stopped at a newsagent on Borough High Street to buy her a newspaper, and at Pret's next door for my own sandwich. We met in Guy's courtyard. The sun shone. It felt as if the summer would never end, as if – this year, for us – time had snagged on an underwater rock, and now hung still; as if there would be an endless succession of these meetings. At one o'clock Nicola would always be waiting for me with a blue headscarf and a cardigan against the cold, and would be with me for one hour – no more – like a princess bewitched, like a girl held captive by an ogre. For a week or two it felt as if time had stopped altogether.

Sometimes, since she died, I've been back to the courtyard to eat a sandwich, sitting on the wall around the grass where office workers chat in groups, and tired-looking nurses lie back and close their eyes to the sun. I imagine Nicola walking along the corridor towards me, head in a scarf, before I return to work. I want to feel time loosen, as it did then; as if it might become so malleable it could even let me back. I want to fall into an enchanted sleep and find myself back in that summer, with Nicola beside me.

I visited again after work each night. On the way home, late, I stopped in the eighth-floor lift lobby and looked out at the City, lights shining in the summer dusk. I cycled home along Tabard Alley, dodging potholes and loose stones. Everyone was away on holiday. On the doormat I found postcards from Greece and Spain. The space in the bed beside me yawned like a grave's mouth. One day I flew up to Edinburgh for work and, high above the Midlands, saw both coasts at once: the Severn to my left, and the curve of Suffolk when I looked eastwards. The plane's engines roared in my ears. I hadn't realised, until then, that it was possible to see everything at once.

Suddenly, unexpectedly, midway through Nicola's second treatment, we found that we were happy.

We were alone together – close together – and at peace. Nothing disturbed us. In the clamorous routines of our lives before illness, we had hardly ever stopped. Our days were busy, full of work, of our family and friends, of people. All that had vanished now. Suddenly we found ourselves alone in fog. Eyes on one another, we took one step forward, and then another. We held hands. We pressed each footstep carefully into the grass, like travellers crossing a marsh, feeling for firm ground. Not once did we raise our heads to look ahead. Nothing mattered but the next step. Living in the moment was cancer's gift to us, in our last year together.

We found ourselves alone on a sea, bewitched. Never had we been able to see each other so clearly. Never had we so clearly registered our own happiness.

Two weeks passed. The last slug of chemo was forced into Nicola's chest line. She texted, *Sleep beautifully my darling and dream about me.* Nicola was young, for a leukaemia patient, and strong. The doctors allowed her home after barely more than a week. She wasn't high-risk, they thought, she would recover by herself. I went to the hospital to pick up her medicines. A plastic bag of strong drugs tugged at my handlebars as I cycled home.

With the chemo working through her system, Nicola's counts ticked slowly down, recording approaching danger like the altimeter of a diving plane. Cavalier about infection, she went shopping, but nothing happened.

Then, one morning when she checked her temperature, the figure in the digital window recorded 37.9. She called the duty doctor at Samaritan. She didn't feel ill, she said, but the doctor told her to take no chances: she should go to A&E immediately.

A&E was the only gateway to hospital admission. To us, it was one of the frustrations of the system: a neutropenic cancer patient, vulnerable to infection, had to wait alongside the urgently sick, and then be sent a mile across London to be treated. I got a text at work: *Still waiting for transport.* When Nicola finally reached Guy's there was no free bed in Samaritan so they put her in the adjacent ward. She didn't seem worried. She texted me to bring in her make-up bag and some soap. It was the last day of July.

'Infections happen the whole time,' said the doctor who came to check on her. 'They might be something you catch in the street, they might be something you already had in you. We all have infections. Our immune systems keep them under control.'

Nicola's immune system was gone, for the moment, wiped out by chemotherapy. We went back to the newspapers and waited for the antibiotics to work. She didn't like being in a strange ward; Samaritan had become home. To pass the time we planned our next weekend away, a treat to ourselves before the third round of treatment. Although they promised nothing, the doctors thought her counts should be back up by mid-August, and the infection ought to be gone by then. Nicola found a hotel and restaurant at Mistley, at the head of the River Stour. It was near where we kept our boat, so we hoped to get a day's river sailing as well. Joe, his A-levels over, offered to come up from London to help.

Days passed – wasted days, so far as we were concerned. Martha sent photos from Norway, where she'd gone for a summer holiday with her boyfriend. Stuck in Guy's, Nicola waited for her temperature to drop, but it stayed stubbornly high. *Hand cream, lip salve, radio lead,* she texted. *More socks, underwear and a dressing gown.* And eventually: *No temperature now.* That night we watched *Nashville* on separate screens a mile away from each other, texting comments on the characters. She finished, *Dozing off. Good night my most wonderful husband, love you so much xxxxx.*

The next day, infection-free, she was so eager to escape they had to lock up her medicine to stop her leaving.

We celebrated freedom with a walk in Greenwich Park. The long view from the hill was full of hurrying clouds. Grass surged over the ridges. We held hands. The wind, scouring Blackheath, smelled of leaves and traffic. We both felt free. Nicola was still tired, but illness seemed treatable. The sun shone as she gripped my elbow. At the end of an alleyway we found a Henry Moore bleached copper green in the bright, clear light. London's horizon encircled us; we felt on top of the world. That was the moment, I think, when we began to talk about what sickness had given us. The solitude it had drawn around us, a close awareness of each other's presence while the world grew more distant; a stilling of background noise; a sense of privacy, like a curtain drawn around our love for each other. Cancer was an eminence from which we could see farther than ever before to a horizon which curved around us in a sharp, distant line. However dangerous the sea, we knew where we were. However uncertain the future, we had clear sight of it. We were as happy together as we had ever been.

The hotel at Mistley was comfortable. Our bed filled a small dark room on the first floor. We walked past a dock closed off by Heras fencing. Abandoned sheds surveyed a narrowing creek pinched between mudflats and a rotting harbour wall. Swans paddled past the buoys marking the channel. At night we could hear the hoot of the Harwich train.

Next day, we went for our last sail together, although we didn't know it then. Joe met us at Ipswich station. We cast off and sailed out through Harwich harbour, our sails filling fitfully in a gentle wind. We turned up the River Stour, heading for Wrabness. Nicola sat contentedly in one corner of the cockpit, reading a book. There wasn't much wind, just enough to keep us gliding past the riverbanks with the tide behind us. We passed Erwarton Point, where once, when our children were young, we would paddle ashore for picnics. They christened the beach 'Whalebone Sands' because of the bleached tree trunks washed up on the shingle. We remembered our friends John and Caroline driving down from London to meet us there. We pitched a tent on the shore and retreated into it when the rain came. Caroline had breast cancer. She died a year later but we still have a photograph of her stooping in the tent, laughing.

Halfway upriver a dredger was manoeuvring. At Parkstone Quays a huge cruise liner awaited passengers. Through binoculars we could see swimming pools and an atrium. Someone, perhaps a sailor, jogged doggedly around an upper deck. Sun gilded the water. Its surface sparkled towards the woods on the far bank, a yacht tacking, two ducks nosing at a buoy. At Wrabness we ate lunch in the cockpit. We couldn't be bothered to pump up the inflatable dinghy and row ashore; we thought we'd be coming back. Our sailing holidays and weekends together had been some of our closest times as a family. We'd watched our children growing up in and out of boats. In the evenings we lit hurricane lamps and played cards in the cabin, while the night drew in around us and the sea breathed the cold salt smell of the marshes. We crossed the Thames Estuary, and out there, between the sandbanks, saw a porpoise leap clear of the water and plunge back into its element, leaving behind no more than an impression of a fin, a shape, a moment of grace.

After lunch Joe and I sailed us home. The wind had strengthened. *Zylippe* heeled in a gust, accelerated; we heard the clop of water under her bows. We knew our children were about to leave home. It wasn't just cancer that was changing us; life always moves on. We'd talked of selling our boat and travelling more. Things come to a natural end. On the reach up to the marina we went through the familiar ritual of furling sails and hanging out fenders, as we had so many times before.

We turned into the harbour entrance, moored, locked up, and drove away. We didn't know then that we'd never go back. When Nicola died, my brother sold the boat for me. My niece turned up on our doorstep one Sunday evening with a plastic box full of our books, charts, cushions, all that was left.

4

It's Christmas now, six months since Nicola died. Martha, Joe and I didn't want to spend Christmas at home. Instead, we've come to Rome. We found a flat on Airbnb. Friends are staying nearby.

I used to know Rome well. Partly, of course, we want to avoid a Christmas that brings back too many memories, and we want to be together. But I also want to be somewhere that anchors me in the time before Nicola, to prove that I haven't lost everything.

It feels the right place to be. There are Christmas trees in Piazza Venezia. Lights sway above the narrow streets, and the shop doors are framed by electric stars. We go into churches, where our foosteps echo from marble, stirring shadows under the arches, and the cold smell of incense. The clunk of a Euro coin in a machine bathes sudden light across a martyrdom, an angel, a pietà. In dark side aisles old women pray. Outside, the streets are full of Christmas shoppers, bars, and little studios where old men carve picture frames, or squint through lenses at antique coins. We climb the steps of the Campidoglio and stop at the railing, looking out over the ruined forum beyond. The wind suddenly feels cold. A dead city, this, in contrast to the living one: broken arches and buried streets, fallen roofs, columns entwined with weeds. Rome stares back at us, half-face, half-skull.

You'd expect people to recoil from all this decay, all these abandoned shops and palaces and temples. Instead, tourists take selfies against a backdrop of ruins. Perhaps we fear death less than we think, or know it better than we imagine. School groups pack the steps of the Trevi Fountain: Russian, Chinese, English, German. Who hasn't lost someone? A father, a daughter, a wife ... Crowds flock in silence along the street that runs through the forums. I imagine each person leading their lost ones beside them, the crowds doubled and redoubled by those we have all lost. Next to Augustus's forum an old beggar, bare-chested, shakes a plastic cup at the passers-by. He makes me think of the old man in the A&E ward at St Thomas's: *It hurts ... it hurts*. At night, gulls float above the ruins, their wings lit white from below.

In most towns, streets join and part logically, and the past is buried. Not in Rome. Here, the dead are entangled with the living, clinging to one another not in archaeology's neat layers, but with the immediacy of an embrace. On a street corner the pavement falls away to expose the skeleton of a shop, unburied, or a dead street where people used to walk. Three columns crumble against the wall of a church.

My thoughts feel the same. I seem to have lost my memory since Nicola died – I can't concentrate; things don't connect. When I think about Nicola and the past year she comes back to me in a mosaic of fractured memories and dislocated ideas that lead nowhere, just like the streets of Rome.

I write in the early morning. As night retreats, the apartment block opposite comes slowly into view: a grey shutter with sagging slats, key stones splaying above a window, a carved lion. Our Christmas tree winks in the corner, and I think of Nicola, the presence no longer next to me; a presence so constant, so vital, it was a part of my own life, as I was of hers; her smell so familiar it was simply the air's smell; her touch, the life pulsing in my own veins; her voice, the clamorous music of thoughts in my own head. We were indivisible, indistinguishable. Waking in the morning meant her weight in the bed next to me; life meant the consciousness that somewhere, perhaps in an office, someone's kitchen, a coffee bar, she was talking, laughing her irrepressible, sweet laugh, her lips widening in her loving, adorable smile.

In the past few months I've gathered all our emails together, all our texts and WhatsApps, and put them in order. I imagine one day I'll be able to make sense of what I'm writing, as an archaeologist untangles Rome, deducing a temple from a pile of stones, or matching a statue to the niche from which it was torn. In any case, all my thoughts circle the one overarching reality, which is the absence beside me.

On 17 August 2015 Nicola began her third course of chemo. It was routine by then. She packed her bag, chose books, folded her headscarves. We had an early supper at home, then I drove her into Guy's.

Her arm ached. It seemed desperately unfair, but she was afflicted with a frozen shoulder that caused her constant pain. Common enough for women of her age, the doctors said; perhaps connected with chemo, perhaps not. We remembered Caroline, the friend we had met at Erwarton Point, hobbling across the grass towards us with a smile, lugging a picnic basket. Chemo had wrecked the joints of her hips. We remembered her trying to play rounders with her young sons, insisting on running from base to base so as not to miss a game which might be her last. But no, the doctors said, this was probably just a frozen shoulder.

All fine, Nicola texted. *Still in remission*.

She was sick, no one was quite sure why, but pills made her feel better. The doctors decided to allow her to come home each evening, until her counts fell. We ate early and I drove her back into hospital, clutching her bag on her lap. Watching her slight, lonely figure disappear into the alleyway that led to Guy's I remembered being dropped off at a boarding school, and the gulf of homesickness and fear that opened up inside me as my parents drove away. I felt bereft, abandoned to a world of arcane rules and routines I couldn't control; robbed of freedom; surrounded by strangers. Nicola must have felt the same. She walked slightly hunched from the pain in her shoulder. She never complained. I sat at the wheel and watched until she disappeared around the corner that led to the entrance.

The only good thing about being apart, Nicola texted, *is the looking forward to being with you tomorrow.*

There was other good news. In America, a friend's daughter was born, and we were sent a picture of a sweet baby in a white woolly hat. Eyes closed, fists clenched: new life.

Things couldn't have gone more smoothly. Horizon lifting, our thoughts turned to the bone marrow transplant that lay ahead. That would be the final stage in her treatment. We weren't sure what to think about it. Some doctors spoke of it airily, as a routine treatment little worse than chemo. Others seemed to suggest it was frightening, to be avoided if at all possible.

It wasn't going to be possible for us, apparently. Dr Clay explained blood markers. One of Nicola's tests had showed positive: an indication that, without the transplant, leukaemia would recur.

'So we'll spin you along to King's,' he announced breezily. 'They'll soon sort you out there. You'll meet Dr Anand.'

We did. She was short, intense and inspired confidence; Nicola liked her at once. Dr Anand explained the principle. Leukaemia is a malfunction of the bone marrow, which starts to produce cancerous white cells. But the bone marrow can be replaced. We pictured a horrific operation, bones cracked open like crabs' claws. It wasn't like that, Dr Anand explained. A donor's stem cells were gathered from their blood. Injected into Nicola's bloodstream, her own marrow would simply absorb them. It was vital, of course, that a donor be found with a close genetic match to Nicola's, or the stem cells would be rejected. Not a relative, usually. There was a database of donors they would search. Many were German. She could introduce us to people who'd been through the process. We booked a date, 11 September, to visit the unit at King's together.

There were risks, of course. The new stem cells would create a new immune system, wiping out the old one like a computer hard drive being wiped clean. For a time Nicola would be vulnerable as a newborn baby.

'You should read this pamphlet,' Dr Anand said. 'It's a bit scary, I'm afraid. It explains everything.'

Nicola was quiet that evening. Dr Anand's pamphlet lay on the bed next to her. She'd been crying.

I sat down and laid a hand on her forehead. 'What does it say?'

'Don't read it.' She pushed it away.

'Why not?'

'It explains what can go wrong. Dr Anand said it was scary. They have to tell you what can go wrong, of course they do.' Nicola shook her head, brushing away fear, and smiled at me. 'I'm going to be fine.'

She had that ability to push worry away from her; she had that strength. I can never 'not worry' about something – worry gnaws me; anxieties wake me at night. But Nicola was able to put things out of her mind at will. It was part of what made her so serene. It enabled her to live through cancer and grow sweeter and stronger with every day. I'd give everything – everything – to change places with her now. For it to have been me who put up with the probings and the needles, the endless pain; the anxiety that never quite vanished, and the terror she felt at night and divulged not even to me. But I would never have borne it so well. Nicola stayed resolute. She knew neither panic nor self-pity; her stoicism was bone-deep. She could spend hours sitting under drips, or waiting on plastic chairs while her blood span in a centrifuge. She laughed off the petty frustrations of NHS treatment – the crossed-wire letters and post-dated appointments – and kept her sense of humour intact. Putting worry from her mind, she did Sudokus, sat on her bed, emailed friends, read detective stories. She was able to banish cancer to the shadows.

And we both knew that this ordeal was not all bad. Yes, we longed to return to normality, but there were things we relished in our new life. We felt all its urgency and freshness. For as long as we were exiled to this strange place, cancer, we felt the thrill of each morning; the thunder of the sun rolling over the horizon; the flare of orange burning the world each night at sunset. Light refracted strangely from walls; the air tasted sour and bitter. And the past had been returned to us. Between treatments I found Nicola turning the pages of photo albums. We recalled holidays we'd taken before the children were born, parties, our wedding, in a detail that had always escaped us before.

With the future out of bounds, the past had never seemed so real. It became absorbed in the present, as if time existed not in a weary sequence, with the present moment running like a bead along a string, but all at once, simultaneously. The day we met felt as real as the consultant's visit yesterday, the pain of giving birth as recent as our weekend sailing up the Stour. No fog hung over our twenty-eight years together. No twilight hid the joys of conversations we had, of places we'd seen, of making love, of being together. The time we'd been given spread out around us, rolling over hills, so broad and wide, so full of incident and life that the tiny moment we occupied – the small room we sat in, the bed, the lamp, the gentle knock as the cleaner stopped her trolley outside, or the monotonous bleat of an alarm from the ward – was merely a cockleshell on a sea; it seemed no more vivid, no more important than anything else. It was just a vantage point from where we could look out over years in which Nicola had not been ill; in which death lay over the horizon; in which the sun warmed our years together, our growing family, our happiness.

The treatment seemed easy this time, a routine. Nurses wheeled in the trolley of chemicals each morning. I visited at lunchtime, and again in the evening. Joe was working in Pret A Manger, saving money for his gap-year trip to America. He'd wanted to stay home until the transplant was over, but Nicola insisted he go anyway. She hated the idea that her illness might stall his life; and so his room filled up with rucksacks, T-shirts and boots. The summer drained away. Nicola came home on 23 August, after just a week. We planned to see friends.

Perhaps we had become too cavalier about immunity. Watching television together on the sofa, on 2 September, Nicola felt something was wrong. She tried her temperature. It was above normal, though not by much. I don't know how she sensed this was more than the usual fever, why she was so insistent that we leave straightaway.

I drove her to A&E. The doctor on duty was young and inexperienced. It was frustrating to have to go through details that seemed obvious to us: Nicola was a blood cancer patient from Samaritan; she had Acute Myeloid Leukaemia; she was neutropenic. The ward was busy so they found us a side room, then left us. Nicola sent me out for water – it was hot. Everyone seemed to be rushing. A harassed nurse refused to catch my eye. When I came back, Nicola snapped at me for almost the only time: she wanted me to push harder for attention. She worried the handbasin was dirty; she worried who had been there before, whether the bed had been properly disinfected. Through the door we could hear voices at the desk, and phone calls being made – none about us. We could see families huddled on chairs at the far side of the ward, a wheelchair being pushed past, and a girl groaning on a gurney, her shoulders covered in sweat. At last a consultant came. Nicola needed to stay in hospital, she said – that we knew already. They were looking for a bed but every ward was full.

They gave Nicola paracetamol to control her rising temperature. Her head ached. The nurse who came to administer the drug didn't know how to use a Hickman line and wanted to put in a drip instead. Nicola dug in her heels until they found someone with the right training. I'd brought sandwiches with us but she didn't want to eat. We swapped texts with Joe, at home. It would be late, the nurse said, before a bed came free.

We waited. Sometimes I went up to the desk to see if there was any progress. From there, I could see into the next cubicle: a girl who was drunk, or perhaps had taken drugs; her family around her. At last an ambulance came. The street was empty. I watched them load Nicola onto it but she wouldn't let me come with her. It was only an infection, after all. I watched the ambulance lurch down the ramp, then walked home along the empty streets.

Before going to bed I texted her: *I hope you're asleep. I'm worried you're getting so weary of it. It really will come to an end. I love you so totally. Xxxxxxx*

She replied, *Would love to be on final stage but it's probably not to be. Temperature spiked again so have just been given paracetamol and hoping for a good night's sleep. I love you so much xxxxxxx*

Before, they'd always managed to kill off infections within a day or so. This one dug in. The doctors tried new antibiotics, hoping to hunt down whatever strain was taking hold of her. A consultant, one we'd never met before, explained, 'Different antibiotics work on different bugs. We try a whole spectrum.'

They took blood, hoping to grow lab cultures that would reveal the nature of Nicola's infection. Sometimes, the consultant said, Hickman lines became infected, so they swabbed the end and took blood samples to see if anything would grow.

Nicola's temperature stayed high. She'd been put on a different ward to start with, but a bed soon came free in Samaritan. That was familiar, at least, frustrating as it was to find ourselves back there. Nurses took Nicola's temperature and blood pressure every hour. Paracetamol brought false dawns of lowered fever, but by evening her temperature always climbed back up again.

I remembered my mother taking my temperature as a child, flicking the glass tube to shake the mercury down, then prodding it under my tongue, where it squirmed uncomfortably, sharp and cold, while I waited for what seemed hours. Nicola's temperature was taken in moments, with a probe in the ear whose plastic cap the nurses could flick into the bin with a single deft movement. We learned the centigrade limits: 37.5 was a temperature, 38 was worrying. Nicola spiked to 39, hair slick over her hot forehead, then 40.

They changed the drugs yet again. One morning, a few days in, Nicola texted, *Had reasonable night but very breathless.* The breathlessness was new. The doctors thought the infection might be in her lungs. That evening, when I went in, I found her wearing a mask that gripped her nose and mouth. Oxygen hissed from a tap in the wall and a new monitor by her bed recorded the level in her blood. 95 was just high enough, the nurse explained. Nicola's showed 88. Nicola tried to grin at me through the mask, but I knew she was tired.

The next evening, arriving from work, I found a doctor in dark-red scrubs reading her charts.

'I'm from the CCU,' he said.

I didn't know what that was. The Critical Care Unit, he explained – Intensive Care. His manner was different from the cancer doctors, who wore shirts and jeans. A stethoscope dangled from his neck. He felt Nicola's abdomen and pulse, and left, promising to come back in a couple of hours.

We tried not to worry. We were glad that quietly, efficiently, they were pulling in extra help around us. The nurses bustled around, tucking in sheets, administering drugs. Nicola's chest laboured under her hospital gown, my brave, strong wife looking ill really for the first time.

A bit shaky but feeling clearer headed, she texted later that day.

I replied from work, *Shall I come?*

No urgency, she wrote.

But that night she was worse. They'd turned up the oxygen. A CCU nurse was examining Nicola when I arrived. Nothing had come back from the latest round of tests, but the air in her lungs was sour and too thin; I could hear the rasp in her throat as she struggled for breath. That evening she didn't want me to go home. I slept on a cold, hard plastic sofa in the unused visitors' room. In the middle of the night the nurse woke me up: Nicola was asking for me. Her hair was slick with sweat and the skin white and taut over her temples.

The duty doctor was short, very young, and nervous. 'We're going to take her down to Intensive Care,' she said. 'It's just a precaution; there really is nothing to worry about.'

A porter stood outside. I held Nicola's hand. I could see a crust of dead skin on her lips. She squeezed my fingers.

'I feel f-fine.' Her voice was fevered.

To move her, they had to unhook the oxygen, then reconnect it to a temporary bottle to take her down to the CCU. But the connector didn't fit. I could sense the doctor getting anxious beside me. It was frightening how quickly Nicola's counts dropped: 88, 86. A technician came. He wrestled with the adaptor. In an American drama this is where the doctor would have bellowed, 'I want oxygen *now*!' Our NHS doctor said, 'Could you hurry up, please?' The technician hit the tap anxiously with the wrong end of his pliers. At last it slipped round, and air gushed into Nicola's infected lungs.

Outside Samaritan they hurried the bed along darkened corridors. The cold blue light of fluorescent tubes shone on anxious, calm faces, practised movements as the bed was manoeuvred into a lift too small for it. Somehow they squeezed me in too. The doctor gave a reassuring smile, then her eyes flicked to the monitor clipped to the end of Nicola's bed. It was bewildering how quickly infection had taken control of my wife's vulnerable body, how contemptuously it had brushed aside the antibiotics. The lift door opened. I didn't know this part of the hospital. We went down a broad, empty corridor. A row of wheelchairs stood in an alcove; we passed locked doors. Nicola's face, labouring for breath, looked small and crumpled on the pillow. We might have been at the top of a tower or deep in the earth's bowels. I was lost.

The door of Critical Care had notices sellotaped over it, warning of infection. Beyond, a long corridor ended in a huge, dark room. The only light came from monitors, and from the computer screens on a square, raised desk in the middle of the room. Around it were rows of beds, each inhabited by a motionless, corpse-like figure. Nobody spoke. I could see an old woman's face, brown against the pillow, her eyes bluish and closed, the sheet pulled tight across her shoulders as if she were in a morgue. Beside each figure, drips hung like teardrops in the half-light.

It felt as if we had walked into an inner sanctum – or a laboratory, the forward station scientists might set up by a volcano, or at the epicentre of an earthquake. We had come closer to death's realm.

They pushed Nicola into a side room, vast and empty, with a space in the middle for the bed. A nurse was waiting. As I watched, monitors were pushed into place to either side of her, drips were hooked up, a line for oxygen connected to the tap in the wall. A new screen winked into life high up on her left. I recognised oxygen level and temperature – 39.9. Her oxygen hovered below 90. I didn't know what the other numbers meant. Nicola lay among the watchful monitors like a sacrifice on an altar. She seemed to be asleep.

'You should go home now.' The nurse was efficient and no-nonsense, more focused and business-like than the

Samaritan nurses, who were disconnecting their equipment to leave. 'We'll take care of her.'

'Is she in danger?' A stupid question: she was in the Critical Care Unit.

'We'll look after her.'

Nicola seemed so small. She looked like the other patients I could see through the inner window. I squeezed her fingers and felt their answering pressure, our lifelong conversation reduced to the touch of finger and palm. I laced my fingers into hers and she squeezed them again. Her eyes, briefly open, still had humour in them. *What crazy things we do together*, she seemed to be saying. I don't think I was scared. It felt like the evening she was diagnosed, a challenge we would rise to together.

'Go home,' the nurse repeated.

But when I left the CCU, I couldn't find my way to the stairs. The lift seemed to have disappeared. When, eventually, I stumbled on the entrance lobby I wondered if I would ever find my wife again. It felt as if some minotaur had stolen her and taken her to his lair.

Nicola stayed ten days in Critical Care. My office was planning its annual trip. I phoned in to cancel and spent the time with her. Until then we'd wanted to keep my work going – it was our way of holding something normal in our lives. It had been hard. It was disorientating to move between a busy office and the odd, sequestered world of Samaritan. When I went into the ward, I felt the sudden, overpowering silence that follows when a machine is switched off. That silence echoed within me as I worked. I wanted to be alongside Nicola as she sat by her window, awaiting doctors or test results. Sitting at my desk I thought of the drip hanging over her bed, of the nurses studying charts, of her fingers stitching away at a tapestry. The people around me felt like shadows; I felt like a ghost. But my being there was our token that we had not altogether been banished; that one day we would return.

Now I just needed to be with her.

'We might beat it with antibiotics,' the CCU consultant said. 'More likely, her own immune system will sort it out when her counts rise.' He was friendly but busy. His expertise was obvious, and reassuring – he had dealt with this before.

I called Martha to explain Nicola was in the CCU, but they had everything under control. Joe came to visit. We settled into a new routine like refugees in a transit camp, used to the uncertainties of life with cancer. In the CCU, hygiene was everything. A poster above the basin taught us how to wash our hands: palms first, then backs of the hands and laced fingers, before finishing by scrubbing fingernails. Infection had been abstract before, now it was real: we had seen what infection could do.

One by one, we identified individuals and families in the motionless patients around us. One came from a Roma community. Her family crowded the lobby downstairs, small men in trilbies and women in headscarves, treating sickness – serious sickness – as a community ritual, a dress rehearsal for death. Vulnerable to everything, Nicola stayed in a room by herself. She had her own nurses, giving 24-hour care in 12-hour shifts. One nurse came from Portugal, another from Wales. We hardly ever saw the same face twice – it was as if Guy's had an inexhaustible supply of nurses. The carers seemed to be skilled in everything: drug dosage, technical equipment, infection control. They changed drips, administered pills, helped Nicola to struggle upright in bed when she needed the toilet, slipped on special socks to prevent blood clots. In their brisk, trained hands, their patients were helpless dolls. Nutrients came from a sagging plastic bag; energy drinks were plucked from a freezer. In a way it was a relief to be surrounded by this constant, slightly impersonal care. There were no decisions to be made. Nicola's body was in the hands of others.

Her venetian blind slatted building works at the back of Guy's. Our radio played on the window sill. When I cycled home in the evenings the air was colder; summer was wearing thin. Nicola was conscious most of the time. Sometimes she hallucinated. It might have been from all the antibiotics she was taking, the doctors said. They told us how most people had nightmares, how they screamed and clutched the sheets. Nicola's hallucinations, by contrast, were benign: a cartoon fox who appeared at the end of her bed, grinning. It seemed there was nothing bad in her for the chemicals to churn up.

As the days went by we got to know precisely, from Nicola's monitors, when the paracetamol was wearing off and another temperature spike rising. Soon it became clear she was getting no worse. The temperature spikes became regular, predictable, and gradually less strong. We followed them on monitors like meteorologists tracking a hurricane that was blowing itself out over a stormy sea. Gradually Nicola's immune system juddered to life again. The storm was past.

She was damaged, though. Her thighs had withered from lack of use. When, at last, she swung her legs off the bed, they were too weak to support her weight. A physiotherapist came. Nicola sagged into a chair, exhausted after five minutes of gentle exercises. When I put my arms around her, I could feel her ribs. Slowly we shuffled from one end of the room to the other, me walking backwards, holding her hands. She was worn out after two lengths. The first time we walked out into the main room, the nurses stood and clapped. Determined, Nicola wouldn't sit down halfway, on the chair the physio pushed behind her: she wanted to make it back to her room by herself. Her face glowed with achievement as she slumped on the bed.

After ten days they moved her back to Samaritan. She was still weak. It would be days more before they allowed her home. Far worse than her lost strength, though, was the damage the infection had caused to Nicola's eyes. Sitting up in bed, she put a hand over her right eye, and then her left, staring intently at the wall.

'What's happened?'

'It's a shape, like Africa.'

Only around the periphery could she see clearly. The centre of her vision was blurred, as if someone had scored her eyeballs furiously with an eraser. The doctors thought there must have been bleeding behind her retinas when her platelets were at their lowest. They promised full recovery but warned it would take time. For the moment, it was like looking through glass someone had scratched with a stylus, Nicola said, or looking in a mirror rubbed with oil. She could see a patch the shape of Africa, beyond which everything swirled and distorted.

I sat on the bed beside her and held her hand. She couldn't read; she couldn't easily make out my face. It was as if the world was already starting to melt and slip from her grasp.

Melting and slipping away – that is how Nicola seems to me now. It's as if we're looking through opposite ends of a telescope at her death: Nicola looking forwards and me back. And in the centre, where our eyes should meet, is nothing but a furious erasure.

It's like that as I write. I can see clearly at the periphery, but the centre is gone. Every time I try to capture Nicola's face, her voice, the result seems so much less than the person I lived with and loved for twenty-eight years. That's the absence in these pages, as it is now in my waking and sleeping life. A blur at the centre, where everything has melted.

I want to find her again. In Rome, when I'm not with Martha and Joe, I walk the streets endlessly, trying to recall her in my memory. My mind keeps wandering. Rome's streets don't lead to Nicola; they just lead to other streets. I'm in a maze. I know Rome but I still get lost. I glimpse Nicola in odd moments. Suddenly I'll find myself thinking about a conversation we had in hospital, or a time we met for a drink before a play. Or I'm sitting in a square – sitting outside a bar while water plays in a fountain and a patch of sunlight lights up a doorway, or a locked church – and she's there suddenly; and then as quickly she's gone again, just as I realise it wasn't her I glimpsed, but a memory of another day, a different moment from which she was absent.

Most of the time I can't think about Nicola at all. I'm like a child peering at the sun through his fingers, seeing pink darkness slatted by blinding light.

Our flat's above a station. The metro rumbles below us. At three in the morning, Rome's rubbish collectors grind through the streets, collecting the day's detritus. At night, my mind runs free, like a madwoman pacing an attic, rummaging the past. I wonder how the earth can bear the twilight's weight, or find energy to hurl the sun into the sky each morning. I need Rome because it is like the whole world, disjointed, but each step I take along its streets leads me further from Nicola. Yesterday it was six months since her death; tomorrow it will be more. I try to look forward but there is no forward. Like a broken aqueduct my life ends in mid-air, spilling water on darkness.

When Nicola came out of hospital after her infection, she was so weak she could still barely walk. We tried to go out on Sunday afternoon. She reached the tower block at the end of the road, then said she had to go back. We took it one step at a time, with Nicola clinging to my arm until we reached the door. At home I made tea. Nicola sat on the sofa with her headscarf pulled tight, a fugitive rescued from a monster's lair.

'We can't do anything now,' Dr Anand said, when we visited the clinic next Monday. 'She needs to recover. The transplant can follow; she needs time. Go away, take some holiday and get some rest. Go away, you both need rest.'

5

The path along the river from my sister's cottage led to the little marina at Woolverstone, a mile and a half away. The first day we went out, Nicola made it only to the stile at the edge of the village. She rested on it, looking at the sunlit field beyond through blurred eyes. The river slipped past to our right, behind trees. Summer had clung on for us. The grass rose up towards a hill, woods, blue sky.

I'd borrowed the cottage in Pin Mill twenty-eight years before, the autumn we started going out. Nicola came to stay. We went to the pub and ate shrimp, looking out over the river, and the hard where Thames barges sat on the flat mud, rusty-coloured sails furled. Neither of us said anything – but that was the weekend, we both agreed afterwards, when we knew something special was happening. Pin Mill was the place our story began.

'That's all I can do.'

'Don't worry.'

'Sorry. We'll do a bit more each day. They said it will take time.'

A dog nosed past us, hurrying onwards to some favourite tree or remembered smell. Its owners followed behind, greeting us cheerfully. We waited while they passed. Nicola leaned on my arm – she weighed almost nothing. Slowly we walked back along the path between tall hedges. Someone was mowing their lawn. To our right we could see yachts propped up on cradles, for sale. I'd wandered through them the evening we arrived. It was lucky the cottage was so close to the hard, a gravel track snaking across the mud where Thames barges moored. At high water the whole bay sparkled in the sun. When the tide went out, the river dwindled to a distant silver band, and yachts lay on the flat mud, masts tilted.

Every evening we sat on a bench with the village green behind us, and watched children play in the stream where Martha and Joe had once waded, making dams. The council had built a new jetty. We watched an elderly couple set off along it to their moored dinghy, carrying hampers of food, a kit bag, oars. That would be us, we thought, in old age. We looked forward to being old together. A man worked on his deck, a ladder propped up from the shingle. Old wooden rowing boats lay on their sides, waiting for the ride to refloat them.

Beside us the sign for Harry King's boatyard peeled in the wind, unpainted. The lights from the pub shone on wet mud. It had been a bargeman's pub, once. Twenty-eight years before there had been an outer snug, where they served beer from casks, and an inner sanctum, a bare, boarded room, where food was served on long tables. New owners had taken it over and turned it into a themed riverside pub with fake barge memorabilia and a ship's wheel hung on the wall. They had turned something real into something that looked real but wasn't. It made no sense to us. The food was edible, though, and the memories strong. Beyond, thick trees hung out over the river, sheltering the houseboat colony whose lights we could see winking through late summer leaves.

'Borrow the house whenever you like,' my sister had said generously. 'It's there. No one's using it.'

I booked holiday at work and picked Nicola up from Guy's, where they wanted blood for more tests. The sun was still hot, early in September. I wore shorts, waiting in the car park on one of the taxi spaces. We were euphoric – we'd won a summer holiday after all. We drove east in dark glasses, listening to the radio. Outside Ipswich we stopped at Tesco to load up with weekend food: pasta, crisps, coffee. The road down to Pin Mill was choked with cars, but when we came out on the river we could see lines of moored yachts swinging to the evening tide and beyond them, thick woods on the far bank, and the green dome of an observatory.

The cottage had just been done up and smelled of fresh carpet. The kitchen was new. We stripped my sister's bed and put on the duvet we'd brought from London. Stooping to look out of the window, I could see a gravel track, and a corner of mud beyond it. We had books, a laptop for music. The next day we drove into Ipswich and bought cheap speakers from Comet, setting them up on the sitting-room floor and playing Roundhouse music from Nicola's iPod and the sea interludes from *Peter Grimes*.

One thing troubled the doctors: the inflammation in Nicola's lungs might have been caused by an allergic reaction to chemotherapy. She would need more chemo before her transplant, but they weren't sure whether it was safe to proceed.

She'd had an appointment with a lung specialist, who X-rayed her.

'The lungs are quite damaged,' he said. 'It'll heal, but we can't do anything yet. It'll take time.'

He wasn't sure whether the inflammation had been caused by chemo or not; he thought not. There was something else, though. When Nicola had first gone back into hospital, as the infection blew up, Dr Clay had come to visit her. He was quite straightforward about it: there'd been a mistake; the dose for the last chemo had been lower than intended. They'd departed from the treatment protocol for Acute Myeloid Leukaemia.

We didn't mind the mistake – we both worked ourselves; mistakes happen. We admired the honesty with which Dr Clay talked us through possible implications. We had a good idea that one of the junior doctors was responsible, but Dr Clay never said that; he took it entirely on himself. He sat on the end of Nicola's bed, with his hands wrapped around one of his long legs. What they suggested was a new kind of test. A unit at Guy's was exploring leukaemia at the molecular level. They could tell, far more accurately than the blood tests we were used to, whether cancer had been banished even from the blood cells' nuclei. If so, there was nothing to worry about. If not, they would increase the dose next time, or maybe plan in a further round of treatment.

'But we can't do anything now,' Dr Anand repeated, in the Monday clinic where we'd done the crossword in a windowless waiting room. 'We need to see the nuclear test. We need your lungs to recover.'

Limbo. We walked along the river at Pin Mill. The sun was shining again. Dragonflies danced above the path that slanted across the field. Today, we'd walked further – Nicola was getting stronger all the time. We knew an opening in the hedge where you could get down to the river, on a flat level of grass with an old houseboat moored on it. From there we could see back into the bay of Pin Mill. Nicola had her headscarf on. A yacht sailed up towards Ipswich, its blue spinnaker tugging it on. It moved fast; the tide was coming in.

'I can see the pub,' Nicola said, looking obliquely towards it. 'I can see the barges, I can't see the spinnaker.' She was looking directly at it. 'A blue patch, just a blur.'

She was stoical, as always, not depressed. Glad to be out in the clear sun, glad to be in limbo. We held hands. The shadows under the trees smelled of earth and crushed leaves; nettles filled the hollows either side of the path. Ahead of us we could hear voices, children. Resting on a log, we talked about cancer. How it had enriched us. How much closer we were now, even though we had thought it impossible that we could ever be closer. We talked about the perspective it gave, how the peripheries of our life had come into focus. The centre, which drained away so much energy – careers, meetings, the daily slog; pressure at work, people being difficult; the rush to get home when a meeting overran, or to a concert or play; the effort to pack in exhibitions or dinner parties when a week's hard work clamoured only for rest – all that had fallen away soundlessly on the day Nicola was diagnosed. We'd barely thought about it since. Other things mattered more: our family, our friends, ourselves.

We talked about working less, perhaps going down to four days a week. We talked about retiring, something that, a year ago, had seemed unimaginably far off. Nicola and I had both been ambitious. We'd both worked hard, assuming that a successful career was the only way to consummate a successful life, the only way to refine energy or intelligence into something usable. It didn't seem like that anymore. The only thing that really mattered was each other. That, more than anything else, filled and illuminated our world. Our love had become the garden in which we lived.

The long, broad river swept calmly past us, a silver ribbon beyond the leaves. Boats drifted on the current. There was just enough wind to stir the water's surface into short, enamelled ripples. Next to the log was a pile of earth where something, a badger or dog, had been digging. We looked out through a fringe of leaves, as if we were in a bower.

'I think I need to go back now.'

'Tomorrow we'll go further.'

From the corner of the path we could see all the way downriver to the cloud of masts at Levington, where we kept our boat; and beyond, to the Felixstowe cranes which stalked the marsh like steel herons pecking for food. I cooked risotto and tossed salad. Music played on the sitting-room floor.

Martha came down for the weekend. We'd warned her Nicola had little energy, and that we were in the mood only for gentle talk. She got that straightaway, and slipped into a quiet mood alongside us. From the very beginning, with her mother's grace, she seemed to have discovered an instinct for what to do, what to say. Like Joe, she could hold fear in check. Love mattered more.

Her presence strengthened us. We walked further each day. At the end of the week, with Martha beside us, we came out on the lawn of the yacht club at Woolverstone. Two boys in wetsuits were rigging a dinghy on a trolley. An old couple sat on a bench, watching boats put off from the slipway. They must have wondered why we looked so pleased with ourselves: a woman in a headscarf and a tired-looking man and girl grinning as they emerged from the trees, as if walking along a river was the finest thing one could ever do.

We found the smugglers' house where a cat was put in the window to signal the coast was clear. The story went that one day the cat ran away and the customs men caught the gang red-handed, and hanged them. Pausing on the way back, sitting on our log, we talked again about how cancer had made us stronger, and happier. Of course we hated it, of course we longed to get past it; but this dreadful year would never be one we locked away and forgot. It had changed us, we knew, for the better. We loved each other more, valued our children more, trusted our friends more. A tide had turned. We felt a contentment in each other, and in the world, that health and good fortune had always hidden from us.

We got a message from Italy. A friend's husband, who'd been diagnosed with terminal cancer, had died.

Summer should have been over, but the hot weather held, the year's final gift to us. I signed out the next week and we went back to Pin Mill. This time we walked east through the woods along the riverbank. The fields had been harvested and we followed a track to the water, clambering over a fallen oak. Under willow trees, at the bottom of a garden, we found a square creek, a secret harbour. Two dinghies floated on it, tethered by sagging ropes. A kingfisher flashed blue across the reedbeds. Lost in weeds, someone had built a cabin there. Peering through the windows we could see sofas, a formica table, a crooked stove: someone's haven.

Another day we went to Shotley, where my father had trained in the war. The old naval base was ringed with barbed wire. Through padlocked gates we could see a parade ground with weeds growing through cracks, and beyond, the fallen roofs of the barracks. The old ship's mast which cadets had been forced to climb looked sad, yards lopsided and ropes rotting. A notice at the bottom warned DANGER. My father, terrified of heights, had forced himself to the top through sheer willpower, and gazed out over Harwich harbour to the North Sea.

We drove down to the marina, where my mother used to take him, during his last illness, for a glimpse of the sea; and followed a path along the north bank of the Stour. Out in the stream the river was a vivid, sapphire blue. The glassy water lapping the path's edge was so clear we might have been in

Greece or Turkey. We could see pebbles lying at the bottom, a patch of mud, an anchor rope trailing out into deep water. Gardens rose above us. We could hear someone's radio playing. Beyond the village we came out on a field with the silver river stretching beyond it, into a distance where water met sky. We stopped at Erwarton, the little dusty-smelling church where Anne Boleyn's heart is buried, and watched old ladies sweep up flowers from a wedding the day before.

When I look back now, this is the month I want to return to; this limbo while we waited for tests and results, more treatment. It floats like a bubble on a stream, desultory yet purposeful, fragile, complete.

In London, Joe did the Guy's Challenge, a fund-raising drive that had him run three times round the hospital grounds, cycle 10K on an exercise bike, then race up Guy's tower. Sweaty but proud, he hugged Nicola at the end. We sent friends a video. The weather cooled.

Walking along the river at Pin Mill, we'd talked about the places that meant most to us. First came London, the city where we'd both been born and lived all our lives, the place we loved most. Then there was Pin Mill and the Suffolk coast; Rome, where I'd once spent a year before going out with Nicola, and where we'd sometimes returned together; and the south-west corner of Greece, Messenia, where we'd often holidayed. And then there was the south-west of France, where Nicola's parents had bought a tumbledown farmhouse in 1974, and where she'd spent her childhood summers. A few years before, her parents had sold the farmhouse and moved to another, an old stone house on a hill. I'd been planning to go out there for the weekend to close it for the winter. Now we realised that, with all treatment on hold, Nicola could come with me.

We flew from Stansted to Bergerac. Driving south, Nicola sat excitedly in the passenger seat, counting landmarks: the church at Issigeac, the rise from where you first saw the castle near our home. She hadn't expected to see it again for months; now it seemed more beautiful than ever. It was as if our world had been remade, in cancer's wake, and offered to us anew. Weeds choked a tumbledown barn to the right of the road. In the little village supermarket we heard the familiar south-western accent. Nicola, fluent in French, had known the area since she was nine. Driving up the hill she gripped the dashboard, peering ahead through her blurred eyes for a first glimpse of home.

The house where she'd spent much of her childhood was a farmhouse among the fields. We'd started borrowing it from her parents the winter after we began going out. We could remember arriving with ice on the pond and hoar frost thickening the trees in the forest behind. There was no heating. We shivered next to calor gas stoves, and burned logs in the huge kitchen fireplace. In the years that followed we returned with friends. Martha and Joe spent their first summers there.

When development threatened the farmhouse, Nicola's parents, Anne and Peter, sold up and bought the stone house on a hill nearby. The track to it wound through trees. Arriving for the first time, we'd glimpsed an old wall, mulberry trees, the edge of a rampart. The house had taken shape in the ruins of a fortified tower. Pigeon holes pierced the walls. Inside the bedrooms, you could hear the cooing of doves. In her years of retirement, Anne had replanted the garden with irises and Solomon's Seal, trained roses up walls. There was a tumbledown shed in the garden where Peter wrote.

We went there more and more as Martha and Joe grew up. One winter we built a new kitchen, Martha sawing sheets of MDF while Joe and I drove to the local town to load the car with worktops and cupboards. We spent Christmas there, hanging paper chains from the beams and decorating a massive tree. In summer, friends lounged by the tiny, tree-shaded pool.

For Nicola, it was the most relaxing place on earth. Reading on the sofa, or in a deckchair on the terrace, her body slid down the cushions until it was almost horizontal, her thoughts lost in George Eliot or Proust. She kept a thick, moth-holed jumper in a chest of drawers upstairs. At night we listened to pine martens under the roof tiles. The view from the bedroom window, when I threw the shutters open each morning, showed a river marked by rows of poplars. To the left were forests. To the right, the rising sun lit up Monflanquin, the local town, as if it were an island village, floating on a sea of mist.

When we arrived that autumn the grass squelched underfoot; it had been raining. As I carried our bag from the car, leaves hung heavy on the trees. The key stuck in the lock. Beyond it we found the house dark, damp-smelling and abandoned. Chairs were shrouded in dust sheets. The fridge came to life with a grumble as we switched on lights. The night we arrived, we ate quietly by the fire from chipped plates and glasses dulled by the dishwasher. Nicola should have been in treatment. Both shoulders ached – the right one had frozen as well while she was in Intensive Care. Her eyes were only recovering slowly. When she turned her head, the cobwebbed shadows of the living room were blurred. But she didn't care. We were in the place she loved best in the world, her realm.

The house on the hill existed outside time. In summer, cicadas shrilled in the grass. Winter hung the trees with hoar frost, and the woods hid castles. Forests ringed the house, impenetrably thick. We knew some paths through them, not all. On long walks I used to tell our children stories about the duke who lived in the castle nearby. When they were tiny we carried them in backpacks; later, they stumped along beside us, gripping our hands and asking what was going to happen next. The trees were chestnut, oak, pine. Sometimes we found mushrooms under the autumn leaves, though we rarely dared eat them. We heard the rustle of wild boar in the undergrowth. A hare lived in the field below the house; buzzards watched us from sagging telephone wires. Each morning I drove downhill to the baker. The midday bell from the local church could be heard distantly across the valley. Nicola's father Peter, a historian, once found out that the commune's population had peaked just before the Black Death. Since then, people had left it in peace. A little shrine by the roadside showed where a resistance martyr had been shot.

Our weekend in France that autumn could have lasted a month, a year. Nicola sat in a lone deckchair on the terrace, reading. It was warm enough not to wear a coat. She smiled when I took a photo. Downstairs, we went through old family albums. Their bindings had split with damp, and mildew speckled the pages. Old pictures slipped from their corners, as we turned each page, or dropped off yellowing sellotape: her mother, younger, beside a 1970s car, with a picnic spread on the verge; Nicola playing by an inflatable pool; or running, arms spread in glee, down the farm track. Time that could not be reclaimed. She'd been befriended by the farmers next door. As a child she'd helped with the harvest, sat on their small, underpowered tractor, fed rabbits. Married, we sat at their kitchen table being regaled with local gossip in an accent I barely understood, while two logs smoked in the farmhouse grate.

Both of the old people were dead now. Gabrielle had poisoning of the blood; his legs were amputated. Renée had died in the old people's ward in Fumel. When we drove past, their house was locked up, no chickens pecking the yard, no small, battered car outside the front door. In twenty-eight years we'd sensed a generation pass. We no longer saw berets in the market, or heard old people speaking dialect. Things changed, even in this changeless place.

On Sunday, Nicola swept leaves on the terrace while I fixed a broken shutter. A year later, when she was in Intensive Care and nearing the end, Martha painted her a picture of the view from that terrace: the little town of Monflanquin on its hill. We taped it to the wall opposite her bed. Nicola lay against the pillows. The tube in her throat stopped her turning her head. I watched her eyes flicker over its patches of green and brown, trees, fields; over the pantiled roofs, the church on the hilltop; over clouds, forests, the cleft of the valley which we knew concealed a river. As she lay on her deathbed she couldn't talk, but I could see her mind think, blurred by the drugs, of evenings we had spent watching the same view or conversations we'd had on that terrace; of the sweet perfume, at night, wafting through the car window as we drove past the green woods

Martha had painted. The week she died, I had the picture framed. It hangs above my bed now.

That afternoon we drove back to Bergerac and flew home.

The blood cancer clinic was held on Monday mornings. Dr Clay's nuclear cell test had never reported back and the doctors were inclined to give up on it. They thought Nicola was probably not allergic to the chemotherapy. She was ready for a bone marrow transplant.

Nicola had been to King's for preparatory tests. Transplantation wiped the body's immune system completely, they told us. The new system generated by donor cells was fragile, incomplete. It had to grow like a baby's in an adult's ageing and unfamiliar body. Any infection was dangerous so there were dental check-ups to make sure no abscess would appear, blood tests, scans. She needed chest X-rays to confirm her lung damage was repaired. There were visits to the Transplant Unit at King's, where she met nurses and saw the isolated rooms in which transplant patients were held.

'People stay in six to eight weeks,' the nurse told her. 'Normally. Everyone gets an infection, though. Everyone goes back in.'

At Guy's we were introduced to successful transplant patients. They seemed shaky on their legs, with the grey faces of the ill, but spoke glowingly of the renewed life it had given them.

'You can live a normal life after a transplant,' one said. 'You really can.'

He and his wife had just been on holiday to Spain, but he'd been hit by an infection and they'd hurried home. Hospital visits would be frequent, he warned us. Nicola shouldn't expect to go back to work for another year.

A nurse read out to Nicola, officially, the list of risks and problems that could follow a transplant, a long list. Nicola signed her agreement to treatment. Next Monday the corridor outside the blood cancer clinic was crowded. We did the quick crossword. They took her 'bloods'. Dr Anand called us in, eventually, to a small office at the far end.

We were only expecting final confirmation that the transplant would proceed that week, but Dr Anand's manner was odd. She seemed both nervous and excited.

'Look,' she said. 'You're going to think we're crazy … I've got some news.'

Nicola sat down. Dr Anand took her hand. Good news? Bad news? They'd found a donor who seemed a good match. Had it fallen through?

'Do you remember the nuclear test we did?' Dr Anand said. 'The one we gave up on? We got the results back – at last.' She cleared her throat. 'It shows there's no cancer in your cells at all. The Professor says patients who show cancer-free don't usually relapse. Sixty-five per cent stay healthy.' While we sat there, still silent, Dr Anand called him on the phone to double-check. His sample was small but the results were clear: Nicola was free of cancer.

'So what do we do?' we asked.

Dr Anand smiled at us. 'Nothing,' she told us. 'Stop thinking about it. We'll check you every month, but there's no more treatment.'

We still couldn't take in the words. A weight gone; a cloud vanished.

'You're free,' she said. 'Go home.'

6

I've changed since Nicola fell ill. I understand sadness, which is the sky I live under. I'm not asking for sympathy; it's the simplest of facts: I'm sad. Sometimes a friend complains how unfair Nicola's death is. I don't understand that. I don't believe some conscious will controls the comings and goings of daily life – who falls ill, who gets well – any more than I believe a God decides, each day, to raise the sun or set the moon. People fall ill. The cancer cells multiplying in the darkness of a stranger's bone marrow have no purpose. They neither single out the wicked, nor allow a cure to someone because she is beautiful, intelligent and good, and because her family loves her. They simply follow their own dizzying, voracious logic, like termites chewing roof beams or locusts shredding crops. The sorrow of Nicola's death doesn't make it unnatural. People die at all ages, and die young not because the Gods love them, nor because they deserve to, but because they fall ill.

I want to say to people: Nothing unusual happened here. Nicola's loss is exceptional to me, Martha and Joe, only because we loved her. Talking to friends a month ago, I said that her death was 'only death'. One of my friends, a doctor, understood: she'd seen children die. The unnatural thing, perhaps, is the horror with which we've surrounded death over the past millennia: the pyramids and burial ships, the angels weeping on tombs; the open-coffin wakes and horses nodding black plumes; the choirs; the women covering their heads with ash and wailing; the Terracotta Army and the slow-marching regiment; the smoke rising from altars; 'The Last Post'. Such terror manifested about an end that will come to all of us; that is no secret or mystery; and that we know in advance is ours. Such horror about the closure we all share. 'She's still here,' we say – I've said it myself. Only in our memories. Nicola isn't here to comment or talk back; to surprise me; to change as she gets older; to change me. Her voice talks in my head only because I knew her so well. She is gone. She isn't in some other place. I will never be with her or see her again. The subject of this book could not be less mysterious: Nicola died.

The miracle to celebrate is that she almost lived. The miracle is in the work of medics who knew what was wrong with her; who knew how the cells multiplied; who knew, from opaque signals in her blood, what end was likely and what might be done to divert it. Who had a name for this malady, and isolated drugs that almost denied its purpose. Who could peer into the cells of Nicola's blood to see their assault massing, and take steps that nearly, so nearly worked. The miracle lies in the generosity of nurses whose life is spent not making money but caring for people who need care; of the doctor whose face reflected our own pain, as we sat in the meeting room of the Intensive Care Unit the day Nicola died.

Reprieved, we left the day clinic in silence. Nicola looked stunned; I was grinning from ear to ear. Afterwards we joked what people must have made of us. What news could make a wife look so appalled and her husband so happy? We sat in a deserted hospital atrium while Nicola called her mother to tell her the nightmare was over. I have a photograph of her writing the note of thanks she wanted to drop in at Samaritan Ward. We had been freed as suddenly as we had been condemned on that awful Friday at the end of May. Perhaps that made it easier for us to believe in our reprieve. The moment of sentencing had seemed unbelievable, too. But it turned out real – and so would this.

I watched Nicola talk to her mother, tears running down her cheeks. Of course, Dr Anand had been realistic with us: a third of patients relapsed; the test sample was small. If leukaemia returned, it could be harder to eradicate, second time around, and it would have to be cleared out before a bone marrow transplant would take. But that was the only drawback; otherwise this was a no-brainer. Walk free now, and, if cancer returned, Nicola could have the transplant anyway. We'd lose nothing. All the doctors were agreed.

I'd asked, simply to explore the question, whether there was any merit in having the transplant anyway, as a double precaution, but Dr Anand had shaken her head straightaway.

'You don't want a transplant unless you have to,' she'd said. 'They're dangerous. The truth is, only 55 per cent of patients make it through.'

Proportions. Statistics. Neither of us had any training in them, nor how to base decisions on them. Once, when Nicola was pregnant with Joe, a test had shown a small risk of birth defects, but the test to eliminate it had carried some risk in itself. A doctor had explained how risks could be multiplied or added. We followed – just – but what we really wanted was this expert, this person who understood the science and had read the research papers, to tell us what he would have done if it was his baby. If he turned out wrong, so be it. Risk is life's essence, its base matter in a world where the future can't be known. We float on an ocean of risk, sailors in a leaking wooden boat staring at horizons clouded by fog banks. Certainty is never ours to demand. We knew experts could judge wrong, but they still judged better than us. And Dr Anand had made it perfectly clear what she thought. She knew what transplants were like.

We walked home slowly. The air dragged around us, thick as honey and sweetly viscous. Cars rolled past, making no sound. I remember a bus stop where we paused to rest. We'd shared so much. Nicola's hand was warm as we climbed the steps home. Her bag echoed when she dropped it on the floor, as if everything around us, the whole sky, had become somehow reverberant, a sounding board for our relief. We held each other. She seemed so small, so warm, alive.

An endless day stretched in front of us, a day we wanted to go on forever, preserving this moment in which everything had stopped. We had lunch at a favourite restaurant in Soho. Nicola sipped her wine. We used, as a game, to plan our ideal day in London. This was our perfect day. But we were too dazed to look at pictures or go to a film, so we texted family, and sent friends an email:

This is to share some rather astonishing news we got this morning. As most of you know, N was due to go in for a bone marrow transplant next week. But her consultant has just got the results of a new, very cutting-edge test they did a few weeks back, and it shows that her risk of relapse is so much lower than previously thought that she no longer needs the transplant, or any further treatment at present.

There is still some risk, of course, so they will monitor her for the next two years; and a transplant can always be done if anything recurs. But as things stand she has no residual leukaemia, and they're telling us she can go back to normal and we can get on with our lives.

We're off to France tomorrow for a few days quiet walking & readjusting to this. But it feels like a good moment to thank all of you for so much support & love since Nicola was diagnosed. More than anything else, that has got us through the past few months. We feel very lucky.

I remember a childhood game: press your hands hard against a weight, and when the weight is removed, your hands float upwards. Runners wade through water to make their legs feel light when the race comes. It felt as if we had put down a bag of stones and could climb a mountain unburdened; as if mist had cleared and we could see valleys, ridges, forests where before there had been fog.

We'd already booked another week in France. We'd planned it as a moment of peace before Nicola went in for the transplant. Instead, we found ourselves contemplating a new life.

Every photo I took, while we were there, shows Nicola grinning. We weren't simply returning to normality; neither of us wanted things to be the same. We faced the future enriched by the knowledge illness had given us: a knowledge of the future's preciousness, its weight and value. We no longer saw time as life's small change. It was treasure to be guarded jealously. We knew where our centre lay.

In France it had become too cold to eat outside. We wrapped up and walked through the forests. We sat in small, dank churches. We lay in bed and listened to the wind. It was five months since we'd dared imagine we would grow old together. That, for us, had always been the termination of a life lived well. Old age together would mean doing the things we loved: reading, travelling, seeing friends. It was the harbour we would enter in good time. For five months we'd been lost at sea. Now lights winked around us in the dark and we were at peace. Nicola's sight would return in time; her shoulders would stop aching. There would be tests and monthly visits to the clinic, but none of that scared us. Risk hung in the air like low cloud, but we both had the strength to live under it. A two-thirds chance of life, after all, was better than the certainty of hospital wards and drips, treatment, fear.

Nicola had been corresponding with a friend of a friend who'd just been through a bone marrow transplant. He wrote of the exhaustion that followed the procedure, of the constant terror of infection, of something going wrong. He was about to go back to work. He seemed like someone fragile in a clumsy world. Something had changed in him: he was afraid. We'd sensed the same from the patients we'd met at Guy's: that transplant survivors were a class apart, grateful for life but at the same time fearful of it, like children with brittle bones. We would have seized that future and embraced it, if need be. Instead we found ourselves walking on thick grass, breath pluming the air, rattling the curtains shut when we returned home, throwing logs on the fire.

Nicola called Marcus, her friend and boss, to give him the good news. He cried. They talked about her returning to work, in no hurry. There were other things she wanted to do. Plans filled the future like cells multiplying in a petri dish. We'd always loved the castle we could see from outside the house. As well as a massive keep, burned in the Hundred Years War, it had renaissance rooms and another wing, more elegant still, that towered over the landscape like a Loire château. Nicola wanted to research the castle and family. Perhaps we would write a book together.

Back in London, she tapped her computer, ordering out-of-print memoirs from local history websites. Jiffy bags arrived from obscure booksellers in south-west France. She'd had no time for that in the months she was ill. All her force of will had been focused on keeping her back straight and her mind clear as the doctors scoured cancer from her blood. Now, revelling in returning energy, she invented a new routine for herself. Each day she went to an exhibition. Goya was showing at the National Gallery. We'd visited the Goyas in the Prado on our weekend in Madrid, just before Nicola was diagnosed. Now we saw them again. Her illness was bookended by Goya: slaughtered rebels, doomed Kings. She lunched with friends. I found her in the study with plans of the castle laid out around her.

When I look back at the texts we sent each other in those weeks they return to the banality we longed for: *Home in 15 minutes. Taking 59 bus from Euston.* And normality closed its doors slowly upon us. With Christmas approaching, we planned our children's presents. Usually we spent the holiday in France but this year, because of the transplant, we'd expected to be in London. We decided to keep it that way, bought tickets for a carol service, and went to Nine Elms to buy a tree. On Christmas Day we crossed the bridge to Westminster Abbey and sat among bemused-looking tourists. None of us was a believer, but we wanted something special: music, the vault soaring above us. Friends shared lunch. Afterwards we walked along the Thames.

I wish, now, we'd made more of it, our last Christmas together.

In Rome, twelve months later, Martha, Joe and I spend Christmas Day alone. We go to the market to buy food on Christmas Eve. As we unwrap presents, a plastic Christmas tree winks in the corner of the sitting room, a present from our landlady. In the evening we go for a walk.

I find I can't look at Nicola's death head-on. I can't get her in focus, seen through the keyhole of her death. I need an artist to paint Nicola, or capture her in a story. I need a room where I can frame her face and go, locking the door behind me, to sit alone with her. Holbein would have painted her with a cat on her knee and a pile of books, a sparrow, a mask of comedy – not tragedy – a clavier. Hockney would have drawn her in Notting Hill Gate, with a poster of Aretha Franklin and the same cat. An artist would know what to leave out, where the essential lay.

Nicola grew up with art. She remembered, as a child, crouching under the table at the gallery where her mother worked, during an opening for one of their artist friends. She grew up knowing that woven into the world was a vision stranger and more truthful than what we see around us. She found it in pictures, in books, in theatre and music: a code unweighted by the everyday; a nimbler way of seeing. Art makes life visible. Nicola knew it as a way of stepping outside the world and finding oneself at its heart. She knew it as sunlight illuminating the fissures in a wall; as a sound heard at night. She knew its failures and its obsolescence; she admired its practitioners for their oddness and courage, and the way they had of understanding defeat. She couldn't imagine a life without it.

But I have no portrait to reveal her. For now, I just glimpse her from one corner of my eye, gardening or reading a book. I remember a way she had of turning her head and repeat it endlessly in my mind, like a looped film. Sometimes at night I hear her voice, but I can never make out the words. Sometimes I think I can hear the shuffle of Nicola's footsteps behind me. The light ahead seems so small it might just be a star, or a distant planet. I feel like Orpheus walking the road from hell.

I try to think of her death but can't. When I picture the past year, it's the unimportant things that stand out. I can remember the blanket they put over her to control her temperature when she was sinking for the last time in Intensive Care. I remember the grassy slope in Ruskin Park where Martha and I sat, one day, while they turned her and changed her sheets. I remember phoning Joe from the hospital car park to tell him he needed to fly home. Our radio shoved onto a top shelf, the dirty table in the coffee shop, the stifling heat outside the Intensive Care Unit while we waited for someone to answer the buzzer. The pens she used for her whiteboard, whose tops got lost in the hospital blankets, the corridor we wheeled her down for yet another chest scan, and the waiting room outside the scanner where Nicola lay, her eyes closed, chest heaving, and a faint, glassy sheen on her cheeks. Domperidone, Fentanyl: the drug names on the syringes that pushed chemicals into her breast.

But when I try to think of Nicola's death – not the moment, but the fact of it – everything blurs. I have to cajole myself into understanding it: that I won't see her again, won't touch her again, won't hear her voice. It's like a lesson taught by rote that I'm unable to memorise.

Yesterday morning, in Rome, I walked to the basilica of San Lorenzo. They were taking a coffin out of the church. The men wore suits while the women wept; two children laughed. Outside were rows of stonemasons, their windows full of patient angels. I feel as if the music that comforts me will soon die away; that the current washing me downstream will come to an end. Routine stretches in front of me like a wooden jetty leading into fog. Nicola is gone. I have to keep repeating it: she's gone.

It wasn't long after we got back from New Year in France that I started feeling depressed. Everything seemed flat. The rising clamour of everyday life was deafening, dispiriting. It was hard to maintain the peaceful clearing we had cut for ourselves during Nicola's illness. Weeds grew over it. I was stressed at work. At home, Nicola played cards. Exhaustion had caught up with her. We didn't go out much, or see many friends. There was less to say to each other; it had all been said in those vivid, dizzying months of fear. I remember coming home from work, seeing lights on in the kitchen, and sensing an absence of the joy I expected. January's dark evenings, sombre and cold. I locked my bicycle to the fence. Nicola turned cards. I cooked, swore when I burned the garlic. When I come home now the house is dark – I would give anything to have those evenings back. At the time, we felt stalled. We still had moments of euphoric joy, but a grey mist drifted across our days.

I knew it was only temporary. I wondered, knowing nothing about it, if I had some kind of post-traumatic stress disorder – perhaps I ought to see someone. Time seemed a better option. Love doesn't flow consistently. Throughout our years together we fell in love, then, when the current slackened, fell in love again. After cancer we needed time to let overstretched muscles relax, wounds heal, scars vanish beneath new skin. We made love again, cautiously, the first time in a while. We looked ahead, booked tickets to France for Easter, planned a holiday in Greece. We talked.

Then, one Sunday at the end of January, we went for a walk round the City. We wanted to visit Wren's churches again. Pushing open the door of St Andrew by the Wardrobe, we were assailed by incense and low chanting. Faces turned. At the altar, a priest in robes raised his cross high; two servers swung censers. It was an Indian congregation, we learned, who used the church on Sundays, when the City workers were gone. The worshippers belonged to the Syrian Orthodox Church, whose history burrowed far back into the first Christian centuries.

We stumbled on the same thing wherever we went. In St Mary-le-Bow we found Egyptian Copts; the Costa Coffee next door was full of murmuring Arabic. All over town, immigrant communities, landing like starlings in a tree, had nested in unused City churches, chanting in Arabic, Aramaic, Greek, prayers that pre-dated London. Gold robes packed in a suitcase, a cross brought from overseas, or a testament whose cracked binding had last been opened in the furious heat of Cairo or Asmara: these were their few belongings, designating home. Incense summoned the haze of Africa into plain white churches with limestone floors, where a brass plaque on the wall commemorated reconstruction after the Blitz, and wooden panels listed the Ten Commandments. The tombs around the congregation were not of their own ancestors but of eighteenth-century parsons or sturdy donors from the City guilds. We were ignored; no one asked us to go. A priest lifted the host. These congregations sought what was familiar in surroundings utterly alien. We felt the same: aliens in a city we thought we knew.

We walked home cheerful: life could still surprise us. And the wonder we had learned to feel was still there, the wonder at every detail life offered: the curve of sunlight on St Paul's dome; two nurses chatting about a boyfriend; a mother pushing a pram. Outside the Tate a street hawker threw bubbles into the winter sun. They drifted across the water and burst on the Thames. The Coptic chanting still filled our ears with strange harmonies. Life was never normal. We went into the Tate and wandered among sculptures and canvases, feeling renewed. Perhaps art's greatest purpose is to be inexplicably strange. Since Nicola died, it's been my greatest comfort. I go to exhibitions, look at pictures, not burying myself in highbrow, but seeking a world abnormal – saints martyred, graces summoning spring – where everything can be seen; where flesh hardens to stone, tears dry, and a woman in a painting can gaze at a sparrow forever.

It was early in February, the eighth, that I got the call from Nicola at work. She was phoning from the clinic. Her monthly test showed something stirring in the nucleus of her blood cells. Her voice was calm, matter-of-fact; so was mine. They were running the test again – one result wasn't enough to go on. But we both knew, we both knew, that cancer had returned; that the storm was rising; that the months of freedom we had enjoyed were just a painted backdrop hung in a theatre, a last wish, a moment of grace.

7

After turning off my phone I looked around the office at people quietly working. I texted, *I love you xxxxxxxx.*

I see now, looking at my phone, that Nicola had sent her text, *Please call when you can*, at 09.51, a whole hour before. I must have been in a meeting. What did she think of, sitting there in the clinic alone? Sixty minutes waiting for my call. We lived through cancer together, but all the time there was a room I never entered, an inner sanctum of fear and despair which she had to brave alone. After her death I found Nicola had been through all her papers, put her will in a folder, closed bank accounts and listed passwords in a file. I don't know when she did it, perhaps during the months when we both believed she was well; or maybe in the fortnight between her relapse and the start of treatment. We both knew how this story could end, but never spoke about it. Nicola entered that sanctuary, bravely, alone.

It breaks my heart to think of it, now, her working at her desk. I wish I could go back and help her with it. I wonder if

I was a coward for not insisting we speak more openly about the possibility she might die. But I know she didn't want that. From me, from her family, she wanted a bulwark to her faith that she would be well. The rest she faced alone.

We knew from the start that cancer had come back. The nurses knew, when we went back to the clinic together, two weeks later. No one met Nicola's eye. It was a long time before Dr Anand called her in. Nicola had just gone back to work, three days a week. I had a photograph of her in her office, grinning, with the Roundhouse in the background. Her team was delighted. They'd managed well in her absence, but everyone had a problem to be sorted or a question answered. Things had piled up. They needed her calm, good-natured, gleeful presence.

Dr Anand drew diagrams on a piece of paper, making nothing much clearer, but the essentials we understood anyway. The nuclear test was the first sign of returning leukaemia. Do nothing and the cells would multiply, as they once had before. *And kill her* didn't need to be said. We faced transplant again, with a final round of chemotherapy to clear her blood beforehand.

Two risks hung over us.

Dr Anand had told us before, though she didn't repeat it now, that returning cancer was harder to clear out.

'Maybe you'll need more than one round of chemo before you're ready for transplant,' she explained. 'Some people do.'

Time dissolved around us. Cancer time. Back to work in six months, or a year? Two years? We had no chart to plot a course on.

And there was another risk as well: last time Nicola had chemo she had ended up in Intensive Care, her lungs infected. Could that happen again? Would chemo trigger it? Was the same infection still lurking in her chest, guarded only by an immune system that we were about to tear away?

'We'll send you for X-ray,' Dr Anand said.

And more tests, and a check-up on her eyes, and an injection in her frozen shoulder. A donor had been found before Nicola's autumn reprieve. There should be no problem, Dr Anand said, in putting the transplant in motion again. She counted back days on a desk calendar, frowning. Final chemo would start on the 29th. We'd booked a weekend in Florence to visit a friend who had lost her husband to cancer six months before. Should we go?

'Of course,' Dr Anand said. 'You need a holiday – make the most of it.'

Nicola had spent her gap year in Florence, learning Italian, but we hadn't been back in ages. We visited churches filled with calm grey columns, cloisters where an orange tree grew in a garden filled with sunlight. It was cold. We wandered through the Uffizi, looking at pictures until Nicola announced firmly that her energy was going. We talked. We watched the mosaics glitter on the ceiling of the baptistery. We knew religion only from old art, we realised, not from faith. In Santa Croce we looked at frescoes of grieving monks, a sorrowing mother. Our friend dropped us at the station.

Nicola and I had travelled throughout our time together, to France, Italy, Germany. We got engaged on the Charles Bridge, in Prague, the year the Iron Curtain fell. We were staying with journalists who came back from the border to report queues of Trabants, roofs piled high with boxes and trunks as families fled to seek new homes in the West. We never managed to go further afield, but Europe we knew and loved.

This was our last trip, though we couldn't know it. Passport control; security. At the gate Nicola rested her head on my shoulder, tired. Flying over the Alps, the clouds below us looked like the hills of an unknown, unvisitable country, a place we would never see together again.

Nicola's fourth round of chemo was harder than the previous ones. We were both impatient to get on to the transplant itself: we had tasted freedom and wanted more of it. We sensed open fields beyond the walls of the city in which we were besieged. Samaritan, Nicola's shabby home, seemed too familiar. The view from the window didn't excite her anymore. Two weeks' treatment, the doctors said, but they kept her in for four. Everyone was worried about the infection she'd had before. Maybe it was still brooding in her body, waiting for chemotherapy to open the gates of her immune system. Maybe she was allergic to the chemicals after all.

If Nicola was scared, she didn't show it. I think she knew, as I do, that the next best thing to feeling brave is to *act* brave. She didn't talk about infection as they took her obvs, stacked pills into her bedside cupboard, inserted the Hickman line that would serve her through transplant. She texted, *Dr Clay about to come and talk to me. Please remember lip salve.*

To start with, they allowed Nicola home in the evenings. When I got back from work I found her waiting on the sofa. I'd cook supper; we might watch a film. At nine we got in the car and I drove her back, headscarf askew, clutching her bag, to drop her at the gate opposite the Shard. As I watched her slight figure dwindle under the streetlights I again remembered being dropped off at boarding school after a break. Homesickness eviscerated me; I hated the regulation, the loneliness, the distance from home. Remembering it all, I wanted to run after Nicola and hug her, but knew I would see her tomorrow. *Darling one, dream of me*, she texted. I replied, *I love you more than you can possibly believe.*

I had a cold. Visiting, I had to talk through a mask. But our love had once again burst into full flame. I can feel its heat now, as I go through texts. *I can't wait to see you in the morning ... Darling one dream of me I'll dream of you ...* At work

I thought about her. At night, alone, I felt her shadow next to me in the bed. I texted as soon as I woke up; at lunch, I cycled to the cancer ward; at six, I left my desk and made my way through the shadowy alleys off Borough High Street to the post where I chained my bike, to the slowly revolving doors of the lobby, the lift, the locked ward door – and at last to the room where Nicola waited for me.

The feared reaction to Cytarabine didn't materialise. A doctor she trusted said he wasn't concerned about the transplant; Nicola had proved herself strong. They were too cautious to let her home, though. I went alone to a friend's fiftieth birthday, and texted selfies to the ward. Infection threatened but didn't take hold. At weekends we walked up to Bermondsey High Street, where Nicola had found a park she liked, with roses, stunted in February, and a bank of grass behind some housing blocks. Some friends took me to the opera. Martha came up from Cambridge to visit.

Joe, meanwhile, was about to set off for America. He had wanted to cancel when Nicola relapsed, but she wouldn't let him.

'You can stay in touch on the phone,' she said. 'Write a blog. You're going.'

Keeping him in London would have acknowledged the possibility she might not survive, and Nicola had banished that thought from her mind. So Joe set up his blog, and went shopping for better shoes, a waterproof case. For his birthday I bought him a camera. Nicola stole my T-shirt to sleep in, and texted from hospital, *Bored*. Her blood counts were down again, responding to treatment, and she spent hours under drips, watching someone else's red blood and yellow platelets slowly invade her veins. She was home for Easter Sunday.

Before her relapse we'd planned to spend Easter in France, but Nicola had left France for the last time after New Year, our wheels crunching on gravel as the house disappeared around the corner of the track. Instead, I cooked spring lamb for Anne and Peter and we drank wine from Cahors, to make us think of the south-west. Late March, I emailed friends:

Everything is going very well here. Nicola has sailed through her preliminary chemotherapy. Despite its strength she had no bad effects, other than tiredness, and they've just re-done the cell nucleus test which shows that she's cancer-free even at the molecular level. So she'll head into her transplant mid-April in the best possible condition.

Unfortunately they decided to keep her in Guy's for most of the four weeks in case any infections transpired (they didn't). But we now have a three-week lull in which to pack Joe off to the States and hopefully see some of you before she goes into isolation for the transplant itself.

Two days later, Nicola's temperature started to rise. It was 4 April; she was due to go in for the transplant on the 17th. Joe's backpack stood in the hall. Time seemed to be pouring away. There was so much we were meant to do in that last fortnight.

We wanted to see friends while we could. After the transplant, we knew, Nicola would be isolated for months. Still more important, we wanted to give Joe a proper send-off – his plane took off on the 6th. Then there were details to get ready before Nicola's long stay in King's, at the Transplant Unit.

On top of all that I'd arranged for building works while she was away from home. Roofers stood by to tear off our leaking gutters, and have all ready for the earliest date she might return. We wanted to use this last fortnight to gather our breath, pull our family around us for the final leg of our long, difficult voyage.

And now her temperature was going up. Nicola sat on the bed, checking the little white thermometer: 37.8. Numbers were our judges, throughout her ordeal: of cancer cells and blood counts; of the oxygen, much later, that couldn't penetrate her damaged lungs. 37.8 counted as a temperature.

Nicola stuck the tube back under her tongue and gave me a dejected look. She didn't want to go back into hospital, but when she called the ward they told her to come in.

It was the usual routine: St Thomas's A&E. This time I didn't go with her, though I don't remember why not. I have her texts from A&E: *I haven't met a nurse yet.* I was due in Edinburgh the next day – perhaps she wanted me to sleep. We swapped texts as I took the train north, went into meetings, ran to Waverley station for my return. After cycling fast to Guy's, I found her in an unfamiliar ward: there were no beds in Samaritan. Her temperature was down, but the doctors were waiting for the results of a flu test. We both worried about the transplant.

And Joe was leaving the next day, while Nicola was stuck in hospital.

He went into Guy's to say goodbye to her. I think about it now, still: the last time she spoke to him. I thought about it then, knowing the risks the transplant carried. And Nicola, of course, thought about it, too, for all her courage, for all the determination with which she insisted he leave. Her son, her youngest child: as she hugged him, she must have known she might be saying goodbye. When Joe flew back to us, seven weeks later, Nicola was breathing through a tube, sedated. When she opened her eyes, it must have been one of the ways she learned how ill she was, that Joe had flown home to be with her.

I took the morning off work and went to the airport with Joe. When Martha had left for a summer in Africa, three years before, Nicola and I had gone to the airport together. That was the moment Martha's childhood ended: our daughter's small figure swallowed by the security gates. On the train home we'd cried together. This time Joe and I sent Nicola a selfie from the Gatwick Express, grinning. His massive backpack teetered on the rack above us. As the train rumbled through south London suburbs, I knew that the door was closing, once and for all, on Martha's and Joe's childhood. Raising children had been the greatest adventure Nicola and I took on together. We never wanted their childhood to end, but of course this moment had to come. If Nicola had never fallen ill, this would still have been a year of change.

At Gatwick, Joe and I had a coffee, joked. He looked so young. He checked passport and money belt; we hugged. On the train I texted, *Left Joe x*, and kept my face turned to the glass so the other passengers couldn't see my face.

Two days later, Nicola was home unscathed. Her temperature had dropped again. The flu test was negative.

She went to King's and reported back on the Transplant Unit: small, clean rooms, friendly staff, a transplant nurse she liked. She signed all the forms, a grisly process where they read out possible downsides and side-effects and made patients sign an agreement. It was like asking prisoners to sign their own warrant of execution. We knew the risks: rejection, Graft versus Host Disease, skin rashes, damaged organs, infection, death. Nicola didn't talk about them. There was only one path ahead, for us, with cancer lurking to either side, and she stepped boldly onto it, not troubling to look back. My wife's last gift to me was her own courage.

Two weeks before, we'd booked a weekend away, but cancelled it when Nicola's temperature rose. We booked again, a hotel in Woodstock, near Blenheim Palace. Driving west, stuck in traffic near Oxford, we remembered weekend breaks we'd taken before. Through the car window we watched trees softening in the early spring. As a child Nicola used to stay with her grandparents in Gloucestershire. We'd both missed the countryside during her illness. Late in life she'd become a gardener. Somehow, without apparent effort, she had learned how to tie roses and prune clematis, how to summon irises, peonies and foxgloves from a flowerbed, conjuring each in turn as if summer, unfolding like music, was her gift to her family. Dressed in faded jeans and flat shoes, she crouched over flowerbeds, with her glasses slipping to the end of her nose, while the binbag beside her filled slowly with weeds. Gardening was something she didn't share even with me. It was the place Nicola went to be alone.

In Woodstock, wisteria climbed stone walls. The hotel was corporate and depressing. We preferred to visit the palace, its vibrant baroque towers and broken pediments rising above the surrounding trees. Baroque, *barroco*, comes from the Portuguese word for a flawed pearl. Nicola and I lay on the bed reading magazines. I hugged her, my flawed pearl. The next morning we walked to the lake. Under the waterfall, we didn't talk about the possibility of her death. Fifty-five per cent of patients, Dr Anand had told us, make it through a bone marrow transplant. There was nothing to say about the alternative; we chose life.

Nicola was due to go into King's on Sunday evening. They would start treatment straightaway. We left Blenheim after breakfast on Sunday morning and drove quietly home. We both wanted to be brave, but neither felt it. The house seemed empty with Joe gone. Martha was still away in Cambridge. We were quiet but there's nothing, now, I wish we'd said to each other: in twenty-eight years we'd played love's every key. Everything ends. Nicola's suitcase was already packed: headscarves, Kindle, pyjamas. She stuffed toothbrush and make-up into a sponge bag while I made lunch. Neither of us wanted a glass of wine. Our talk was forced. We remembered grey Sundays in the old days, when shops were closed and streets empty, and there was nothing to do but go for a walk or watch an old film. I could feel time unspooling. Two o'clock. She didn't want coffee.

After a silence, she said, 'We might as well go.'

So I picked up her case and we walked out of the house. Now, I want to freeze that moment as I locked the door. I want that afternoon back, cold as it was: Nicola quiet beside me, the trees still bare. The hollowness in her voice when she spoke, the way she cleared her throat on the steps.

I started the car, drove slowly down the familiar street where we'd always parked, turned left. We drove south under the plane trees of Camberwell New Road. Traffic grumbled. We found a parking space on a side road opposite the hospital and walked in through the gates.

Men stood on the steps, smoking. Families were leaving as visiting time ended. The hospital was vast, impenetrable, but Nicola knew the way. We walked down a long corridor with ward names marked on wooden boards. The Transplant Unit was buried within another ward. We rang the outer buzzer and waited. I remember a metallic voice from the entryphone: *We've been expecting you.* It was like something from a science fiction movie. Inside, canisters of oxygen lined the corridor. There were no windows; we might have been in a spaceship. The doors to either side were marked INFECTION RISK.

Nicola's room was on the left, past a further set of doors. It was hot. They'd been sterilising it, the nurse said. She said, *sterilisin'*, her accent unplaceable. The unit felt hushed; there was none of the cheery clatter of Samaritan. Rolls of protective aprons hung on the wall. Faintly we could hear nurses talking in a side room. It was early evening but the lights were already dimmed. A porter rolled a trolley of dirty plates past Nicola's open door.

'I'll bring you the menu later,' he said.

We took stock. The usual bed, but the blankets were different. Everything was cleaner, newer than in Samaritan. A black anglepoise hung over the bed like a butler waiting for orders. A fridge perched on a table, muttering quietly to itself.

To one side was a huge shower room. I stacked books on the window sill while Nicola unpacked her sponge bag and folded tops and knickers into the cupboard. The last patient had left their calendar on the pinboard: foals in a field. A television filled the wall opposite the bed.

There was a brick wall a metre from the window. I could barely see sky at all, and we couldn't hear London. There was no phone reception. Anything could have been going on outside the walls of this place. You could imagine a park, a village, or the shore of an island; a prison yard, a garden, or a deserted city with homes abandoned and shops boarded up. We felt like convicts or fugitives: like Anne Frank in her attic, or a prisoner in the condemned cell, watching twilight through the bars.

I left Nicola at ten and drove home. The builders were due to start on the house next morning. I texted friends:

Keeping you all in the loop – Nicola was packed off last night to King's in Camberwell for her bone marrow transplant, with some preliminary chemo to suppress her immune system to the right level. She'll be in 4–6 weeks. We didn't get to see many of you in the gap after the last bout, because a minor infection unfortunately hauled her back into Guy's for a few days – nothing serious. But we did get a lovely weekend in Oxfordshire, photo attached. Meanwhile, all is going well. The room is comfortable, and the doctors fantastic.

This is all very much routine for them, so we hope this is the final leg of a long marathon.

8

It's New Year's Day in Rome. Last night we went out with friends. At midnight we stood on the Campidoglio and watched fireworks over the forum. People lit paper balloons with baskets dangling below them, carrying wishes scribbled on scraps of paper. We watched them rise into the air. Dozens of candles, man-made stars, they drifted above us, dipped, and burned out over the ruins. A flock of gulls, disturbed, wheeled over us. I didn't much want to talk. Walking home we pushed through New Year crowds: lovers and wives, families with children.

In an odd way, coming to Rome has prolonged the strangeness of the year Nicola was ill. Everything here is strange. I open the shutters each morning, and looking to the right, leaning on the cold marble sill, I can count the ruined columns of the Forum. A broken tower rises at the end of our street. In a church nearby are the chains that bound St Peter's hands. Nothing makes any sense. My wife, my children's mother, is dead. But at the same time, everything is sharp in my memory: the year we had together; the Snapchats we sent every day; the quiet room in which Nicola died, her forehead warm under my lips.

I hate that we've started a year Nicola never saw; that never saw her.

At King's we settled into a new routine. Guy's was just round the corner from where I work. Now I had further to go. Leaving at six, I cycled furiously into the wind. Tail lights jammed Camberwell New Road. I always felt late. For some reason that bicycle journey to King's has left a scar on me. Most of the time, I'm fine. I can work confidently all day, laugh, joke, run meetings, but when I get on my bicycle to go home, I find tears running down my cheeks. A friend, also bereaved, said, 'It's because you're reliving the journey. I used to drive to the hospital. I cry in the car.'

The route soon became familiar: the right turn by a solicitor's office, the railway bridge, the hospital looming above me. There was a cherry tree that started to come out in the weeks I cycled past. It blossomed and was over by the time Nicola died.

Arriving, I ran up the hospital stairs, washed hands, wrists and thumbs, wrestled into gown and gloves, and spent all evening with her. We watched *Scandal*, an American series, then fell back on old favourites. We were halfway through *Bleak House* when they moved her to Intensive Care; I haven't finished it yet. In the days running up to the transplant Nicola felt well enough, except that the chemo designed to suppress her immune system made her sick. She hadn't been sick before; it seemed unfair. I listened to her retch in the bathroom, then gargle and come out smiling.

They allowed her out each morning – so long as her counts were high enough. She went for walks in Ruskin Park, and texted me photos of flowers coming out. It was spring. There was a tree she liked to sit under, a copper beech. The first weekend, she showed me the pond and the bandstand with a proprietorial air, and we sat under her beech. Ruskin Park isn't big; we walked round twice. The hospital chimney glinted in spring sunlight. Some geese had just hatched by the pond, and waddled importantly over tarmac, shaking their yellow fluff. A judo class practised on the bandstand. Down by the allotments, a notice was wired to the fence proclaiming a 'Community Garden'.

Someone in the nineteenth century had laid the park out. The trees were mature, but everything around them had declined into shabbiness. Weeds choked the formal garden. The horse chestnuts in the avenue were overgrown. It felt like the magic garden in a children's book, as if it had been closed up for years. We paused under rhododendrons, thick and dark. Parrots shrieked overhead. There was a path through long grass that reminded us of our river walk at Pin Mill.

Some years ago the park had become a hangout for addicts, the nurses told us; now they were trying to clean it up. The boating pond was dry, with long cracks scoring the cement. From the high ground you could see all the way across London: the Shard, the City and Eye, the housing blocks at Loughborough Junction. Nicola and I stood and looked at the view, hand-in-hand. We would never leave London, we'd promised each other years ago: it was our town.

At home I stood on the roof discussing rafters and plywood with the Romanian builder. You could see miles from there as well: Big Ben, the Elephant and Castle. Our bedroom ceiling wept dust. The rot was far worse than we'd feared, but I wanted everything done before Nicola came home.

'Four to six weeks,' the consultant had told her. 'Three weeks would be a record.'

Dr Anand was off the ward, working in the lab, but her colleague, Professor Lake, was brisk, kindly and expert. There was a well-defined protocol to transplants, it turned out, with prescribed doses and timings that seemed slightly military. We were at transplant minus nine, they told us, the day Nicola went in. They didn't tell us the name of our donor – British, they said, though many came from Germany. It wasn't a difficult procedure for donors. They simply gave blood, enriched first by stem cells leached from their bone marrow through a course of injections. We'd met one patient who'd been to visit his donor in Düsseldorf. He and his wife had wanted to thank him, he said. The donor had become a family friend. Selfishly, we just longed to get past the transplant and out the other side. We wanted our old lives back.

Transplant minus six. We watched *The Durrells* at weekends, dreaming of Greece; read Joe's blog from New York; saved up *High Society* for Sunday night. It was the closest we could get to our Sunday-night ritual of a TV movie at home. I got used to the shop where I bought Nicola iced tea and newspapers. I learned the twenty-four steps to the first floor, where there was a door marked Cardiac Endoscopy, with an old patient in hospital pink always sitting outside it. The menu at King's promised much, but the cooking was as bad as ever. Nicola retched into her toilet. I cooked food for her at home and brought it in Tupperware. On Saturdays I pushed a trolley round an unfamiliar supermarket in Camberwell, loading it with biscuits, crackers, processed cheese. At home, the roof was off. I slept downstairs. Each morning, builders tramped through the house, leaving muddy footprints on the carpet. Rot had wormed its way deep into the timbers, we discovered. We stripped back slate to expose papery plywood, blooms of mould. Everything had to be hacked out. Above us the sky was blue and cold. At night the builders spread tarpaulins in case of rain.

The transplant was planned for 26 April. Nurses counted Nicola down through prescribed doses of chemo. They raised bottles to the light, intoning her name as they checked it against their lists, as if we were commencing an ancient rite. On the day itself I left work early and cycled south. The Anthony Nolan Trust, who'd found the donor, sent a card wishing her well. Nicola was excited: this was the treatment that would cure her. I took a photograph of her in bed, smiling.

This morning I scrolled back through photographs of Nicola on my phone: photos of her in Guy's just after being diagnosed; photos on our weekends at Penshurst Place or Mistley; photos at Blenheim; photos of her in France; pictures of her sitting in bed, with a blue hospital curtain behind her; or curled on the sofa at home; photos of her walking, resting, raising a glass. In all my photographs she's smiling, her mouth wide and eyes alight with fun. Her headscarf might be askew and her glasses crooked; she looks tired, in some of the pictures, and thin; but illness never robbed Nicola of joy. It never quenched the love she felt for me, for her family and friends, for life. Her eyes, in photographs, are brighter than the eyes of the living. Amused, cheeky, full of affection. Glinting with the joy of these lost moments, a joy she retained while the rest of us grew fearful, while her body rebelled, while disease crept up on her from behind.

At six o'clock the transplant still hadn't arrived.

'They come late, sometimes,' said Jen, the transplant nurse. 'Don't worry.'

We worried. We didn't want any hitches. We'd got this far; now we wanted it over. To lose the day, to become keyed up again for tomorrow, was more than we could bear.

Emails were sent; the transplant was in transit. Evening faded on the brick wall outside Nicola's window. We watched *Scandal* and talked, not about the transplant. Guy, the friend who'd been through it, had said it was an anticlimax, 'just a blood transfusion.' He got a bad reaction, but they controlled it with drugs. 'The worst thing,' he'd written, 'is the fear.'

At last Jen knocked on the door: the courier had arrived. We watched her set up tubes and cables, call another nurse to double-check her obvs. She bowed over Nicola's Hickman line, screwed in the connector.

'There.'

Dark blood filled the tube. A first drip shook the bag, quivering the taut plastic; the timer on the monitor winked. It had begun.

'I'll check you in ten minutes.'

We played cards. It would take three-quarters of an hour for the enriched blood to flow into Nicola's veins, for the ritual in her body to begin as old cells were slaughtered and new ones absorbed. I pictured bees circling in a hive. I knew it wasn't like that – this was cutting-edge medicine, wizardry that saved lives. Jen popped in and out. Nicola's temperature stayed flat; it was, indeed, an anticlimax.

But both of us felt exhilarated. This was the cure, the game-changer that would pull her out of cancer's reach, a lifeboat rescuing her from the sea. We knew we faced some long and difficult years, but at the end of them lay health, normality. We knew that Nicola's immune system would be destroyed. For a time she would be naked, exposed. But absorbed by her bone marrow, the new stem cells would start to build ramparts of their own against disease, infection, bacteria.

'You'll have to have your childhood vaccinations again,' Dr Anand had told us. 'Polio, MMR, that sort of thing.'

We joked how Nicola's donor would be younger and healthier than her; she would end up a superwoman. To start with, Dr Anand told us, her immune system would be like a child's. She used a striking phrase: 'a fledgling'. We'd watched fledglings on the trees in France, blinking at the world, testing new wings. Scrawny and vulnerable, they hunched on branches. When Nicola's hair had grown back, tufty and irregular, she'd looked a little like a fledgling, blinking as she woke up. Once she'd been elegant, but she stopped dressing smartly when she fell ill. Instead she wore comfortable old trousers, too-large cardigans and T-shirts she stole from my drawer. It was as if she didn't need elegance anymore.

I think that in illness Nicola became everything she could possibly be. Her bravery, her kindness, her genius for love were all there, all part of her. Dying, they took on a new richness and warmth, like the colours of a painting deepening with the passing of time. I said in the speech I made at her memorial that Nicola was not just more gifted, but had fewer faults than anyone I ever knew. She wasn't petty, or jealous, defensive or insecure. She wasn't resentful, moody, anxious or vain. She didn't know how to hate or carry a grudge. Contentment steadied her. She looked past storms.

Love glowed on the water around her, like light shining from the portholes of a ship. Somehow Nicola forged through trouble, unperturbed. By instinct she dismissed anything negative. She had the intellect to know what mattered, the strength of will to stick to it, the humour to laugh through difficulties. She had the generosity to live for other people, the purity of judgement to know what and whom she loved. All that was there, throughout her life. In illness, her perfections came into focus, lit by a setting sun. Nicola was generous and gleeful, wise and mature. She knew not to complicate illness with fear. She knew how sorrow could house joy.

On transplant night she lay in bed as the blood dripped into her system, eyes already closing. It was late. Jen had stayed on past the end of her shift. It was half past ten by the time she packed the drip away. I kissed Nicola and cycled home. Transplant Day. I was keeping count, at home, of the nights she stayed in hospital, Xs marked on the squared paper of an old notebook. She'd been in nine days; I circled the tenth.

Four to six weeks was the norm, after a bone marrow transplant. Nicola bet she'd be out in three.

'It's a waitin' game,' Jen had said.

There was nothing for us to do. Professor Lake came round each day. Her team followed behind her like the goslings in Ruskin Park. Blood was drawn daily for tests. Nicola still felt sick; they changed the meds. Joe blogged from Birmingham, Alabama. We couldn't go out of doors. While nurses changed sheets or checked dressings, I wandered along the ward to a waiting room whose windows surveyed the park. The cleaners went there too, on their breaks, lounged on the blue plastic banquette, made calls in fast-flowing West-African French or slow Jamaican. A television blared daytime game shows. After leaving Nicola each night, I went to supper with friends nearby. I was more scared than I admitted, even to myself – I can see that now. It felt odd sitting at someone's dinner table without her.

But she was doing well. I've got a phone video from 2 May, transplant plus six, of Nicola and I dancing next to the bed. Martha spent weekends with us. We watched *Pride and Prejudice*, the eighties series with a glowering Colin Firth. Nicola stayed cheerful. Like a top exam student, she seemed to be sailing through transplant with no points lost. She would be one of the lucky ones – she felt no bad reaction, no exhaustion, just the sickness which had started with chemotherapy. I baked rolls and brought them in a blue plastic bag, concocted picnics of supermarket taramasalata and Babybel cheese. We ate them on the end of her bed. She spoke on the phone with Joe in New York. The Trump election was gathering pace; Joe went to a Bernie Saunders rally and heard Bill Clinton speak.

It was a waiting game.

On 4 May I was up in Edinburgh for work. As I landed at City airport I got a text from Nicola, *I've got news*. I called in panic but she wouldn't tell me what it was.

'No.'

'What's happened?'

'It isn't medical.'

Scared, I hurtled down the escalator, ran from platform to platform, leaned over the handlebars of my bike. I made it from the airport to King's in forty minutes. Nicola was sitting up in bed, grinning. A letter lay open beside her: she'd been offered an OBE for services to the arts. I hugged her through the trailing cables of her drip. The letter was on stiff, yellowish paper, satisfyingly old-fashioned; it looked as if it had been typewritten. We speculated who might have put her up for it. I promised to call the number on the letterhead next day, to say she wouldn't be able to collect it until autumn at the earliest, even though things were going so well. Nicola had friends who had turned such awards down – *Empire?*

Really? That didn't even cross her mind. It was an award, it was fun, and her parents would be delighted. She'd rung them already, swearing them to secrecy.

Next, two weeks in, I came in to find Professor Lake standing by Nicola's bed, beaming. Her white cell counts indicated that the transplant had 'engrafted'. I pictured the booster of a space rocket cutting in, thrusting it towards terminal velocity. A new star in the sky. There was no sign of any infection.

At home, Adrian finished the roof. He worked all weekend to do it, just in case they let Nicola out.

'She'll probably go home on Monday,' said the junior doctor on duty that weekend. 'But Professor Lake needs to sign it off.'

I pushed furniture back into place in our bedroom, hoovered the stairs, made the bed, then went round the house spraying taps and doorknobs with disinfectant. I pictured Nicola's fingers touching light switches, opening the fridge. She would be home soon, and it was still only three weeks since she went in. Transplant had indeed been an anticlimax. We wondered when she would be allowed to go to theatres and cinemas. I texted, *My darling love sleep deep and sound. I wish I was there to hold you.*

The next morning her obvs showed a temperature, a small one.

Her bones ached, too. Not badly; the doctor thought it might be a reaction to the chemo. Neither of us worried too much. We wanted to break the record for coming home, but we had time in hand; even another week wouldn't hurt.

But by Wednesday, Nicola's fifty-first birthday, her temperature was worse. I gave her a Japanese bowl I'd found in a gallery on Marylebone High Street, but she wasn't as enthusiastic as I'd hoped. She wasn't feeling well. She was tired, too, more tired than before. And the nurse on duty was bothering her. It was important to take paracetamol early, to stop her temperature spiking, but when Nicola rang to ask for her dose, the nurse took forever to respond.

Professor Lake sent her for a chest scan. It was precautionary, she said, just to make sure nothing worse was going on. We didn't sense worry among the medical staff. Hadn't we been told transplant patients went from infection to infection? It was never going to be a straight road. All the same, both of us were disappointed when the next weekend came – four weeks after admission – and Nicola's temperature was still spiking.

'We'll change the antibiotics,' Professor Lake said. 'We can try something stronger.'

She spoke about taking out Nicola's Hickman line, a possible source of bugs. Tests were sent off to the lab, seeking to isolate the strain of infection.

We couldn't stop thinking of the previous autumn, when a chest infection had landed Nicola in Intensive Care. Now her chest felt tight again. Standing by the machines, taking obvs, the nurses told her to take deep breaths. A new monitor was wheeled into place to track her oxygen. I went in each morning. Good days brought elation. *Am awake and feel much more like me*, Nicola texted on the 15th. *All oxygen, blood pressure etc steady overnight tho I did spike a 39.9 temperature at one point. Have eaten a banana and am practising breathing. Call me when you wake up. I love you.* But a few hours later her temperature rose again.

We could tell something was going on inside Nicola's body, but didn't know what. Like soldiers trapped on a hilltop, we were being outflanked. Although we didn't know it, these were the weeks in which death took up residence within her. We saw nothing; our eyes were on infection markers and temperature spikes. We didn't see – no one could see – the gradual hardening of her lungs; the chaos in her blood; her immune system, panicked by intruders, turning against her own body. The process was as deadly, as impersonal, as an avalanche sliding down a mountain. It was no one's fault. The human body isn't a machine, mass-produced. Nervy as a wild animal, high-strung and fragile, each system reacts differently to the same drugs. Nicola's decline was triggered by forces that were never fully under control, and never could have been.

A week after her birthday they took out the Hickman line. They found pus at the end of it. Everyone hoped we'd traced the infection to its source.

'I think we've turned a corner,' the weekend doctor said.

Nicola smiled from her bed. She wasn't getting up anymore. Sickness made her tired; it was easier to stay in pyjamas. She'd given up completely on hospital cooking, whose smell nauseated her. I left the office early to cook her food, but she didn't have any appetite. Sickness wasn't a problem in itself – she would get over it as the chemo wore off. But it made her feel weak and demoralised as her temperature rose and fell in the first two weeks of May.

The autumn before, antibiotics had cured her. We waited for the familiar magic to work, for the temperature spikes to become less severe and the infection markers to go down. The doctors adjusted her drugs. It was still less than six weeks since Nicola had gone into hospital. She was still in the 'normal' band. Although it was annoying not to be the star patient anymore, there was nothing to worry about. The next weekend we watched *Singin' in the Rain*. Hope came and went. On Sunday she had a better day and we breathed a sigh of relief. It felt as if a corner really had been turned. But her fever spiked again that evening.

'It's never a straight path,' the doctors said.

They'd seen this before. Normally, things worked themselves out. But Nicola was becoming tired, I could tell.

She had less energy for movies or books. And for the first time, she was starting to feel scared. One night she called me at eleven. A nurse from the ward next door had been sent to look after her. He wouldn't listen when she asked for sickness medication – he said it wasn't written on her form. He wasn't experienced with transplant patients. She didn't feel safe.

I got in the car and drove to the hospital. Nicola was distressed. The nurse was an older man. He became defensive when I asked – as tactfully as I could – if her medication was under control. I walked through the corridors, looking for a doctor. Eventually someone came, a quietly spoken young Sikh, who read her notes under the anglepoise lamp.

'You can trust this nurse,' he said softly. 'I've known him for a long time. He knows what he's doing.' His voice carried conviction. He talked calmly through the treatment, spoke to the nurse and adjusted the meds. When he had gone I sat with Nicola for a while, in darkness, hoping she'd get some rest. Outside, orange light glinted on bricks. Her dressing gown made a dark shadow on the back of the chair. It was like the first night she spent in hospital. I didn't leave until she fell asleep.

Another week passed, and still Nicola's lungs closed up imperceptibly, like the slow squeezing of a fist.

I texted from work as often as I could. Her replies always tried to reassure me. She'd discovered memes and sent me a heart. Three ducks in a row was a private joke to reward the list of completed tasks I'd sent through: laundry, shopping, her lunch cooked. At home I washed and ironed headscarves soiled by sweat. Visiting, I sat in a chair, trying to stop my eyes glancing to the temperature gauge. Inexorably her temperature rose every six hours as the paracetamol wore off and the next spike gathered. Sweat blurred her forehead. Her hand, when I held it, was warm.

And gradually her breathing became more laboured. One evening I came from work to find her lying in bed with a plastic tube in her nostrils. I wasn't panicked; neither was Nicola – she'd been given oxygen when her lungs were infected before. We listened to air whistling in the plastic tube. After a while the doctors switched from the tube to a mask. A nurse in dark-red scrubs squeezed a new machine into the room. It had a water tank to moisten the oxygen and stop her nostrils drying out. Nicola smiled at me through her mask and waved her hands. The nurse in red came from the Intensive Care Unit, we were told.

She came again, later in the evening, and this time brought an ICU doctor with her, a burly man with bare forearms. Suddenly we felt closer to the medical coalface; he brought with him a whiff of blue lights and emergency, and his manner was blunter than the gentle academics in the Transplant Unit. He filled the room, too big, an intruder.

'Maybe it's an infection, maybe it's something else, perhaps GvHD. The truth is we don't know,' he said abruptly.

Graft versus Host Disease. We'd been warned of it in the run-up to transplant. It meant the donated cells had attacked the host as an enemy. We didn't want this to be GvHD. That would mean something had gone wrong with the transplant, our lifeline to safety. We wanted it to be an infection which – surely – they could cure. Another day passed. Nicola didn't seem to get worse. At lunchtime I rushed home to cook her lunch and brought it in a box to King's. But she couldn't eat it, and threw up after a few mouthfuls.

It was the last meal I cooked her. That night I read aloud to her from an old crime novel a friend had given us. I left the book on Nicola's window sill with her glasses, the bag with her tapestry in it, the DVD for *Bleak House*. Back home I found a text on my phone: *Debussy and Chopin. Great way to end the day. Sleep well my darling xxxxxx.* At 02.06 I woke up suddenly, aware my phone had been ringing. There was a missed call from the hospital. When I rang back, they told me Nicola's breathing had got worse; they'd decided to take her down to Intensive Care.

The streets I drove through were quiet, as if the city was in mourning. Tarmac shone orange under the streetlights. A burglar alarm winked over a shop. I parked in the empty car park. Further down the road, an ambulance stood with its doors open, a red blanket on the gurney inside. There was no one in the entrance lobby. I wasn't sure where Intensive Care was, but on the corridor leading to the Transplant Unit I met Nicola and her doctors coming down: two porters slowly pushing her bed with a drip swaying over it, a nurse carrying a bag.

Her headscarf had come off. All her hair had gone with the last chemo but one forelock clung bravely on, dark against her pale skin. Her head looked small on the pillow.

She squeezed my hand. 'I'm fine.'

Nicola was always a wonderful patient, wanting to reassure the doctors, to be no trouble. They wheeled her on, the bed slightly askew on its castors. We turned left at the lifts; a nurse held open swing doors; we rolled down a ramp. Inside the ICU, they pushed her to one corner of a long room framed with beds, and asked me to wait outside. I sat by a desk where a nurse tapped a keyboard, her face lit by the computer's glow. The door behind the desk was the room where Nicola would die, five weeks later.

'Would you like a cup of tea?' the nurse behind the desk asked.

I said I didn't want anything, looked at the lino floor. We'd been in Intensive Care before; Nicola would be cured again. I thought of Pin Mill, of walking along the river, past silver water screened by trees; or resting on a log, talking. Nicola's frail body getting slowly stronger; walking a little further each day.

At last a nurse came down the corridor. 'You can come and see her.'

Nicola lay in one corner. They'd put her sponge bag and glasses on a shelf. In the bed opposite her an old man arched his back, muttering. Around us I could see rows of patients. There was a desk where doctors and nurses quietly worked. Calm purpose filled the ward. Although I didn't yet know its name, we had arrived in the Frank Stansil Critical Care Unit, a place we would grow to love. We would get to know Carly, the nurse who looked after Nicola that first night. Months later, she came to Nicola's memorial. We were in the place where Nicola would die.

The consultant had a gentle, precise and high-pitched voice, sounding words as if he were playing an instrument. His hands were large and white.

'We'll see how she does in the morning.'

'I'll stay with her.'

'We have visiting hours.'

'I need to be with her.'

'Call in the morning and you can talk to the matron.'

They left me alone with her to say goodnight. We whispered so as not to disturb the other patients. I found a hand under blankets and wires, and squeezed it. Nicola seemed reassured to be in the CCU. Last time everything had turned out fine.

And she remained as strong as ever. 'I'll be fine. You need to get some sleep. Go home.'

'Are you sure you're OK?'

'Of course I am. Go home.'

Nicola was the thread that tied my life together. She was its tide, the bedrock under its soil, its dawn and dusk, its animating light. Our home was silent and cold, as it is today. Everything that mattered to me lay in that bed. She *was* my home.

I squeezed her hand one more time and left.

In Rome, I've been thinking of that first night in Frank Stansil. I've been thinking about my years with Nicola. I suppose I must be damaged by what's happened, but I don't feel damaged, just tired.

I've tried to think about my future without her.

I imagine that after this earthquake I'll build again among the ruins – a dwelling house in one corner of what was once a palace. I'll use its broken walls for shelter, like an old man in a shed, the caretaker. The past will be littered about me: columns, a plinth that once held a statue. I'll be a guardian of memories. Mounds in the earth will mark out walls, corridors, rooms only I'll remember. I'll recall a fountain, now dry, when water gushed from the mouth of a vase held by a little boy; I'll remember a painting of a girl playing with a cat. I'll cut weeds, chase crows away. At night, in my memory, I'll close my eyes and tell myself it was true: there was once a palace here. Opening drawers, I'll find scraps and odd relics:

perhaps the keys to an old car, or the blanket one of our children lay on. So much has been lost. My head is a museum to a forgotten way of life, housing memories in rows, with a basement filled with shards that don't quite fit.

I don't feel sorry for myself, I feel shocked. I'm like a tree struck by lightning. Only spring will show whether leaves sprout again. I'm like Rome, a city of ruins with a living city around it.

Sitting outside a bar I scroll through photos of Nicola on my phone. I watch us dance again beside her bed. Zooming in, I can almost see her smile. This New Year has helped. Rome is so old, it makes me feel it's not just me that's tired but the whole world, built over, destroyed, and built again. Yesterday I went to an old church whose columns were gathered, during the Dark Ages, from different ruined temples. A building constructed from fragments of ruined buildings. And it struck me that my life with Nicola was the same. We didn't invent happiness but learned it, pilfered it from lives around us. Cities aren't built from scratch; no more was our life together. Our life was old before we lived it. Love was old before we fell in love.

Our story has been told before and will be told again: a man and woman fall in love and have children. One day the woman gets lost in the forest and doesn't return.

A friend said, not so long ago, 'You've lost so much.'

All stories start with someone getting lost.

9

There was a picture of Frank Stansil outside the ICU. Martha, Joe and I used to wait in the lobby for hours, looking at it, while nurses and cleaners bustled around inside. Everyone was too busy to answer the door. Phones didn't work in the Frank Stansil Unit. We made calls on the broad staircase that led to the lobby and even there, ear pressed to the only window, the outside world seemed remote, its inhabitants talking through static like astronauts.

We *were* the world, and in a way, it's still like that. I don't think I've quite left the room where Nicola died; her skin warm when I touched it, taut over her skull; the mole that appeared on her right temple after she got sick; her wide mouth; and the machines that couldn't save her fallen silent as if in sorrow. All our lives together we'd found havens from where we could see everything, like ships on the sea. That's what our marriage was. Frank Stansil was the last of them, and despite its being ugly, the curtains faded and the lights fluorescent; despite the blue plastic chairs stacked in one corner, and the rows of monitors coloured beige; despite all of that, it was the right place for Nicola to be.

It was a beautiful place to die in. Frank Stansil was the most humane place I've ever known, a place of kindness and hope, of learning, skill, wisdom. Outside, the Brexit vote was a month away; demagogues urged people to ignore experts. By contrast, Frank Stansil was a living embodiment of enlightenment, a community of the sick and the generous, of the knowledgeable and those who needed their knowledge. Machines stood in the corridors like an extension of human reason, fashioned to capture our bodies' turgid malfunctions, to analyse, cure and heal. I've never, before, been to a place where expertise was so natural, or so respected; or to a place where people were treated so equally, levelled by their own imperfections.

The next day, the consultant, a new one, took me into his office. Nicola was very sick. Her lungs, he said, had been 'horribly damaged'. It was impossible to say why. His office was a room in which many people had been given bad news. I asked questions whose answers should have been reassuring. Could lung damage heal? It could. Was there still a prospect of long-term cure? There was; it would take a long time. The consultant's manner was less reassuring than what he said. It was as if he was trying to impress on me what I already knew – that Nicola was very ill. Perhaps he mistook my optimism for a refusal to face the truth. I knew perfectly well Nicola was in danger. But he didn't know what it was like to go through a year's cancer treatment. We were used to danger; it didn't seem as frightening as before. And he didn't know Nicola: that, to her, there was never any point in contemplating defeat. Hope mattered more than anything, and we still had hope.

They needed a better scan, 'to see what's going on'. He used the analogy of lungs smoke-damaged after a fire. I pictured soot and inflammation, like the photos we were shown at school to put us off smoking. They needed to send a camera down her throat, but they couldn't do it yet; she was too frail; she had to be stabilised first.

'She's been sinking for a few days. You can see the pattern.'

We hadn't seen it; we'd been too intent on watching her temperature. At her bedside a new nurse, Anne-Marie, cheerfully took control of dosages, monitors, pills. I was in the way.

'You should talk to the matron about visiting hours.'

In those first few days in Frank Stansil I read the insistence on visiting hours as bossy hospital regulation, and fought it. It took time for the penny to drop: we all needed time out. Families and carers needed to recover as much as the patients did. We all had a race to run.

In the next bed a man lay with his eyes closed. They'd been trying to wake him for days. His wife stood over him.

Sometimes she played a tape of their daughter's voice: *Daddy, it's me.*

I sat in the corridor while they changed Nicola's sheets. She was cheerful that first morning, exerting herself, once again, to beat illness with sheer spirit – and to protect me. Since dawn she'd been deluging me with texts: *R u awake? Xxxxx ... How about avocado mozzarella and tomatoes for lunch ... And shortbread ... I am completely wrapped in wires ...* She texted a photo of her pyjama'd legs with cables trailing over them. *Are you like a puppet with strings?* I texted. *More like an escapologist,* she replied.

I texted a photo of Martha sending her a hug, one of my favourite pictures, a daughter's love and kindness caught on the screen. Our friend Nettie was staying from America. I sent a snapshot of them having breakfast. *People sending you waves of love.* Marcus called from the Roundhouse. I'd spoken to Joe on the phone the night before. Now I telephoned Nicola's mother to let her know about the move. *I've got a personal nurse!* Nicola texted, and a bit later, *Impressed! Prof Lake and her team just been to see me ... About 100 doctors floating around ... Come back ASAP!!*

I emailed friends:

A quick update: Nicola sailed through the transplant itself, and all the early signs are that's gone really well. The last fortnight's been a bit harder, though.

She's been hit by an infection which is proving very stubborn. They're currently keeping her stable in critical care, which is giving them a chance to investigate further, so they can target whatever's going on. As you can imagine, Nicola is being incredibly brave and stoical. On the plus side, they're now in a position to work out what's wrong, and already have some good thoughts about what they can do to sort it.

Sedation was the doctors' proposal to stabilise her. They needed to relieve her tiring lungs. The consultant explained it to us: they would put her to sleep, then 'intubate' her – pass a tube down her throat to help her breathe. It shouldn't be there for long, he said, perhaps 24 hours. The long-term aim was to wean her off oxygen support, get her breathing fully for herself.

It was afternoon by then; I'd been there all day. Martha was with us. Nicola looked from the nurse on one side of her bed to the consultant on the other, then to me and her daughter, standing at the end.

'Sounds great,' she joked. 'Send me to sleep and I'll wake up well.'

Of course we knew she was in danger; so did she. I asked if we could have a moment together. We didn't say goodbye – that would have been admitting how near we were to the edge, to darkness, to silence. We were sure she'd get better. Martha kissed her and went out. I held Nicola's hand. We didn't say goodbye, because that would have been too final; but we managed to, somehow, in our own way. That was the moment we told each other, in words we'd used so often before, but were never stale, how much we loved each other; what our life together had meant. *I love you*, repeated again and again. She said, *You're everything*. I said, *You're everything*. I went out. The team was waiting in their green scrubs. Martha and I went for a walk – down the stairs and out through the atrium, along the corridor, into the bustling street. People walked past, unknowing. The gates of the park were open. Beyond the weeds, the leaves of Nicola's favourite tree spread over the grass, casting shade. We sat on the log. *You're everything*. They were the last words she ever spoke to me, or to anyone.

Something went wrong. Nicola's body teetered on the edge, fragile, vulnerable. If it had been a machine, red lights would have been flashing, systems shutting down. Not even the doctors knew how damaged she was.

The aim was for them to carry out the endoscopy – put the camera down her throat – after a good night's sedated sleep. Then – we'd mapped the road ahead – they'd know how things were, track the infection to its source, find the right drugs – and all would be well.

I went to work, attended meetings, glanced endlessly at my watch. I pictured Nicola's eyes closed, sleeping quietly. As soon as I decently could, I left and cycled to King's. I half-fantasised they'd have her awake again, the star patient. Instead, she lay on the bed, shrunken. Her lips were parted, gripping a thick plastic tube. Her hands hung limp.

'Did you carry out the test?' I wanted good news.

The consultant took me to his office.

'She isn't strong enough,' he explained.

It would be the first of many such conversations. He explained how ill she was. She had reacted badly to the intubation, or maybe had just lurched downwards last night, like a sinking ship shuddering as water pours into its hold. They hadn't judged her strong enough to bear the procedure.

His face creased in concern. 'I have to tell you ... she's really not in a good place.'

I stayed calm. An instinct: panicking never helped. I needed to help them help her, not get in the way with panic or fear.

'OK,' I said slowly. 'So ...' I hesitated. It mustn't be the end of the road. But there was something else on my mind. I would need to tell Martha and Nicola's parents how things were, find a way to break the news that things were worse. And then there was Joe.

I said, 'There's something I need to understand. This is my decision, but I need your opinion. Our son is travelling in America. I have to decide whether to ask him to come back.'

I was asking, *Is she going to die?* He didn't answer, quite – he obviously thought it was crazy we'd let Joe go away at all. He didn't know Nicola.

He moistened his lips and said cautiously, 'She's very ill.'

Martha was sitting by the bed, holding her mother's hand. The day slowly passed. From time to time we went out to the park, buying tea on the way, sat on the grass and sipped it. Parakeets flew between trees. In the daytime there was no one in Ruskin Park but drunks and mothers pushing buggies. We talked. Martha and I had been very close when she was a child. Lately, as she grew up and found a boyfriend, we'd drifted away to an adult distance. Now we talked freely again. Her cheerfulness was like a drug. She was like Nicola – so strong, all her instincts full of sense, positive and kind. I wondered how we could ever have been so lucky to have such children. Later, I went out to the hospital car park to get a signal. It was 7am in Los Angeles. The phone droned. I watched porters help an old man into an ambulance and held the phone to my ear.

'Dad?'

My son's voice from the other side of the world. Above me pigeons breached the grey clouds over Camberwell. I told him calmly that things were not so good. I said, 'I think it's probably best if you come home.'

'OK.' He didn't make any fuss, ask questions. I didn't have to say, *Your mother may die.* He knew what I meant; its nuance; our hope. He was in LA railway station, just arrived.

'Can I go online, find you a ticket?'

'Leave it, I'll sort it.'

'Money?'

'I'll call when I've found a flight.'

He was just nineteen. His voice sounded stronger than mine. An hour later I got a text, *Arriving tomorrow, 11.15.* I still don't know how he did it. Around me, when I'd rung off, visitors parked cars; nurses arrived, bags slung over their shoulders; two women smoked on the bench by the steps.

Meanwhile I called Nicola's mother. She was matter-of-fact as always. 'Can she have visitors?'

'Of course. But she is asleep.'

'I know. Peter will want to see her.' *To say goodbye*, she didn't need to say. We made arrangements, rung off. She'd been so strong, like her daughter. I went back in. Nicola was lying unchanged, Martha beside her.

Martha said, 'I think we should talk to her. Maybe she can hear.'

We stood either side of the bed, stooped over Nicola's pale forehead and closed eyes. And this was when we started telling her stories about our life together, our shared memories, the things we had done.

Martha said, 'Mamma, do you remember the time we drove back from the village in France? The car windows were open. It was summer. We played music.'

I said, 'And there was the time …'

It was hard to keep my voice under control. I don't think I'd ever cried in front of my children before. One after the other, we described times we'd been sailing together, birthdays, evenings at home. Large memories and small, we turned them into stories for Nicola. There was no sign she could hear. Her eyelashes, thick and dark, fluttered, like a trail on the surface of calm water as a dolphin turns beneath. Perhaps she was following us down London streets, or chasing some thought of her own, a fleeting memory disconnected from ours; or perhaps it was just drugs stirring in her body, churning up silt.

The nurse moved quietly about her work, checking flows, changing canisters of chemicals. She didn't want to disturb us, but she listened too. Around us, behind curtains, the other patients slept, lost in their own worlds. Our voices grew hoarse. We were both tired, but not as tired as Nicola, my wife, Martha's mother.

Words had always been part of our life together. Nicola knew how to turn the world into words, so it could be shared. At her memorial, her friend David gave a beautiful speech about the conversation Nicola had brought into his life. By 'conversation' he didn't mean anything artificial or forced – quite the opposite. He meant her skill at turning life into a flow of words to be shared: words facetious or profound, words that conjured up people, that plumbed the depths of ideas, that allowed new ideas to be born into the world. Words had always flowed between us as we sat in her hospital rooms, waiting for treatment to end. We'd talked since the day we met, but never so much as we did in that final year. Sometimes silence fell – we were good at being silent together, as well – but more often we filled the hours with talk. It wasn't that we knew our hours were dwindling; neither of us expected Nicola to die. But hours were precious in this new world where everything was precious. Words mattered.

Nicola couldn't speak, now she was sedated, so we filled in the words for her. Stories had always been part of our lives. On long car journeys we read books to each other. We told stories to the children each night. In France they slumped on the sofa to listen to *Black Hearts in Battersea, Mortal Engines* and *The Thief Lord*. Everyone listened. The house in France was a place made for stories. On long walks through the forests I told the children tales about themselves, and the adventures they had. They always started by getting lost in the woods, or missing the path, or being caught in a storm. All stories start with someone getting lost.

For Nicola we turned our own life into stories. I found myself telling things in order, trying to disentangle holidays we'd taken; the year we moved house; the year she changed jobs. It was like finding an old album in a chest of drawers, or a kite string tangled one afternoon and left behind for others to unravel. I didn't know so many years had passed. The past had dust on it; we gently blew it off. Brought back a sunny day on the river; brought back a winter in France, snow, ice thick in the puddles and a pond that creaked when one of the children put a red boot on it. Stories we'd told at Christmas; stories about the past.

Outside the ward I heard Anne's voice: she and Peter had arrived. I don't want to write about their visit, which is for them to remember alone. Martha and I waited outside. I checked my watch, pictured Joe at the airport – he'd have six hours to kill. He had an uncanny knack for travelling. Once, still young, he'd been on a week's sailing course. Stormbound in the Channel Isles, he had somehow found his way home, and turned up on a quayside in Essex with his backpack, aged thirteen. He had an extraordinary self-sufficiency. His travel blog, which Nicola and I had read while she was on the Transplant Unit, had been a joy. We hadn't known he could write – perhaps he hadn't realised himself. His words, beautifully crafted, carried all of his irony and wry humour. His intelligence was of a different kind to Martha's fierce, terrifyingly quick intellect. He slipped through the seas more quietly, watching and understanding.

I wanted to be at home when he arrived; Nicola was unchanged. I showered, then stood at the kitchen window, waiting. A bus came, pulled away, and left him bowed on the pavement behind it, stuffing something into his pack. When he stood up he looked older. He'd grown a beard. It was a man who hugged me on the doorstep. He'd only been away seven weeks. As a man he'd sit beside me in hospital, by Nicola's bed or in the consultant's office as we were told, week after week, that she might die.

'Are you OK?'

'I'm fine. Let me take a shower, then I want to get down to Mum.'

I was so glad to have him back. I held him close, a strong body – not someone I had to look after. We would look after each other, and have done, all three of us, ever since.

At King's he stayed with Nicola while Martha and I went to the park. He and Nicola had last been together in the ward at Guy's, when they said goodbye. He'd always been close to his mother. Our children are like her in different ways: Joe has her green eyes, Martha has her smile.

The next day the consultant said, 'It's touch and go. She seems stable, at least, which is a good thing.'

He sounded surprised how strong her body was. They hoped to be able to carry out their test after all, he told me. I'd lost track of days by then, of exactly how long we'd been here, buying tea, walking to the park, whispering memories into Nicola's silent ear.

Visiting from upstairs, the transplant consultant, a new man, said, 'On the plus side, only one of her organs has failed, her lungs. Everything else is looking strong.'

On the last day of May I wrote to friends, the longest message I'd sent them:

Some of you have picked up that the last week has been difficult. N seemed to be stable, but her breathing got worse while she was under sedation. That was midweek, I don't quite remember which day. They've got things under control, though, and she's now stable and slowly recovering. On the downside, Nicola's lungs are damaged, and the recovery process is going to be very long. The important thing, though, is that they do expect a full lung recovery. And the immune reaction is itself an indication that the bone marrow transplant has worked. So the long-term prospect of having Nicola fully healthy and back to normal still holds as good as ever.

Martha and Joe are both here. We're sorting out the garden for when N comes home.

That was a comfort. Martha disappeared into flowerbeds. Joe and I dug out the edging to the lawn, something Nicola had wanted for ages. Side by side we laboured. Joe hammered in rusty lawn edge with a mallet, while Martha pulled out dandelions and nettles. It was so wonderful to have Joe back; for the three of us to be together.

I suppose we knew this was the unit we might become.

After Nicola died – the day she died – we drove to Greenwich. Leaving the hospital is something I can't think of now. We drove to Greenwich, went into the park and walked. We set each other's tone. All of us cried, a bit, but never at once; the others linked arms and talked on. We knew how we wanted it to be, after Nicola: the same.

Behind us in the hospital, we knew, they must be clearing her room, wheeling her bed away. We didn't think of that; we climbed the hill. Nicola and I had walked there together, between two bouts of chemo. From the top you could see for miles: the curve of the river, London stretching away as far as the eye could see. June, a sunny day, the trees in summer leaf. We walked round Blackheath, had lunch. Walking as if everything was ordinary; so that everything might go on being ordinary, as if our feet on the pavement were the treadmill that turned the world. As if raising a fork, nodding, turning an ignition key were enough, in fact, to create the appearance of life, even when life's spark had gone out. Seeming brave is nearly as good as being brave. To comment on the Observatory, just as we always had, was enough to keep the Observatory there; if we stopped, darkness might fall. And even if one of us felt puppet-like, an automaton, the others were there; other people were always there, passing us on the drive, scolding children, calling their dogs, to let us know it wasn't only us; the world was held aloft by other hands too.

Nicola didn't die – not then. Her head cocked slightly sideways on the pillow, oxygen kept whistling in her tubes. The nurses turned her. We sat around the bed, squeezed her hands, whispered memories in her ears like ambulancemen breathing air into an accident victim's lungs. The doctors were pleased and surprised.

A new consultant called us into the office. 'We're hopeful,' he said cautiously, as if hope was a stick we might steal, like puppies, and run away with. 'We can do the endoscopy. We think there's a decent chance we might have a go at waking her up tomorrow. Perhaps the next day.'

They managed their endoscopy. I waited at work for the results. Nicola's lungs were in a terrible state, they showed: inflamed, scarred, heavy with fluid. The doctors had a better understanding, though, of what had happened. An infection, probably; but then an immune system reaction on top of it, her new immune system attacking her own lungs and destroying them. But the visiting transplant team were positive.

'She's engrafted. Her counts are good.' And they repeated the transplant consultant's line: 'Only one of her organs has failed.'

And lungs, in time, renewed themselves, we'd been told. Months in Intensive Care lay ahead, at best. But that was better than the alternative. There was still a place, a place we could get to someday, where we could be together again with our life restored – or at least some part of it.

We were with Nicola when they woke her up. I held her hand. We took turns on either side of the bed. Her eyelids flickered and I felt slight answering pressure. We talked to her. The nurse moved behind us like a server at Mass. Then Nicola looked at me, her wonderful eyes, green and brown, unchanged. She saw her son; knew then, confused by drugs, that she had almost died; made a face at his beard. I watched him hug her. Martha cried. From the car park outside I called Nicola's mother.

When she was properly awake we explained to Nicola what had happened: the lost days of sedation, the thick tube in her mouth. Another drug had joined the array of antibiotics and antiemetics pumping into her line: Fentanyl, an opiate stronger than heroin. She needed it to tolerate the tube. It didn't seem to muddle her too much, though. The dose was terrifying but lower than usual, the doctors said; some patients remained virtually asleep. We asked Nicola whether she'd heard the stories we'd whispered to her. She shook her head. Only Nicola could have smiled through tubes and a mask. She squeezed our hands, gave a thumbs-up sign – the tube didn't stop her communicating. Her face, always so expressive, could frown, look peeved, shine love on all of us. It could nod at the doctors, thank nurses, or answer their questions with a look: *Good, Bad, So-so.*

Later that day two porters trundled her into a room of her own. She had a nurse to herself, on a twelve-hour shift. It was that much work, keeping her alive. We got to know them all: Anne-Marie, Carly, Naomi, Andy. I wish I could remember every name, every kind face, every pair of gloved hands expertly disentangling drips, or tapping a keyboard as doses were adjusted.

Nicola's new room had a window that looked onto an atrium. Double-glazed, you could hear nothing through it. Her bed was flanked by drips and monitors. A high screen in one corner showed green and red numbers that revealed the secrets of her blood like a survey ship mapping the ocean floor. There wasn't much room for anything else. Her rings had been taken off; her radio went on a shelf in one corner. A bed table carried the few possessions she'd been reduced to: her phone, her glasses. She couldn't read anymore, or manage an iPod. All her energy went into recovery, all her strength into clinging to the cliff face. Her nurses played the radio sometimes, but their friendly chatter was her entertainment in the shrinking world she occupied, an island threatened by rising water. Everything was sterilised, each morning. A curtain round the door was drawn when they changed her bedpan, or replaced tubes. Outside was the trolley where the doctors met each morning, labouring over charts and scans like astrologers reading the future in stars.

While they consulted, we waited elsewhere. We avoided the crowded visitors' room. Usually, while the doctors worked on her, we went down to the coffee shop, or up to the park. We showed Joe Nicola's favourite tree, walked him round the bandstand and pond; the goslings were growing up. One afternoon, at home, I found Martha painting on the kitchen table. She was making a watercolour, three-feet wide, of the view from the terrace in France: the hills, the little town of Monflanquin with its church and tumbling roofs. She painted it on eight sheets of A4. We blu-tacked them to the wall opposite Nicola's bed and put up photographs around it: Martha and Joe as babies; a day out on the beach; her parents; me.

Looking round, we saw tears in Nicola's eyes. In the days that followed she used to rearrange the photos sometimes, so she didn't get bored. She pointed to the pictures she wanted to replace, frowning when we got it wrong. Most of her time was spent propped up, just looking at photographs: her family, the life she so loved.

One of the nurses brought in a chart to help us communicate. We'd point to vowels or symbols; Nicola would nod or shake her head. It took forever. There was a hierarchy of needs. *Is it about how you're feeling? Are you in pain?* The very roots of speech. Seeing how frustrated we were by pointing and nodding, one of the nurses found a whiteboard and some pens. Nicola grabbed them and scribbled busily. Green ink came off on the side of her hand, staining the sheets, but she didn't care. At last she could communicate properly. *Is my mother coming today?* As soon as we'd read each line, she snatched the board back, impatient, and wiped it with the side of her hand. Words erased, just like words spoken, are lost. I wish, now, I'd kept everything she wrote. The only time I photographed the board was near the end of Nicola's life. She'd written on it, *I feel v. positive and also content. I love you.*

We met Nicola's consultants two or three times a week. To start with I met them alone, but Joe wanted to be there too. He wasn't a child to be protected; he could see this was a trial for all of us equally. From then on he and Martha came in with me, and we sat side by side. It became a weekly ritual: the bad news when a new consultant took over at the start of the week, looked at the scans and read her charts; and then their growing confidence as they gauged Nicola's strength. None of them ever gave up: they believed, as we did, in Nicola's tenacity. And her sweet nature spread through the ward. Nurses wanted to care for her. They loved her smile; her gratitude and interest in them, scribbled on her board; and Martha's and Joe's friendliness, so like hers. The Frank Stansil Unit became Nicola's final home.

Early on, we'd hoped recovery might be swift. I think the doctors hoped so too. Nicola was young. She'd pulled through the initial immune system attack, and steroids seemed to have it under control. The aim, long term, was to wean her off oxygen and ask her lungs to work harder as they recovered. There was talk, even, of removing her breathing tube in a day or so.

It didn't happen. Recovery was slow. So instead, the doctors proposed a tracheostomy: to cut a tube into her throat for breathing.

'She'll have her mouth back,' the doctors explained. 'But she won't be able to talk – the tube goes through the voice box.'

Before the tracheostomy could happen, though, Nicola needed to get stronger. It took two weeks. On the day after she texted me, *Tracky likely to be tomorrow*, I was nervous all morning, frightened the procedure would be cancelled again. But when I got to the hospital, Nicola smiled at me – really smiled, her mouth free. Her neck was swathed in dressings. I kissed her, very briefly, on the lips. Her eyes said everything.

The consultant, that week, was inspiring. Energy fizzed around her. She'd decided to take Nicola in hand. After the usual caution at the start of the week, she'd become convinced of her patient's strength and spirit. She was constantly in and out of the room, adjusting the machine that controlled Nicola's breathing, quizzing the nurse of the day about her oxygen levels. It would take time – we knew, by now, it would take time. But Nicola could recover, slowly, cautiously – we were sure of it.

Every night, when I reached the hospital, I got an update. Often I arrived at handover time, just as her nurses huddled over the trolley outside her room, passing on details of meds and observations. Martha or Joe would usually be there, or Anne. But I always insisted that Nicola and I have half an hour to ourselves before she went to sleep.

It was her favourite time, she wrote on her board. And mine too. We got the nurses to wash and prepare her, change drugs, take obvs. They tiptoed around us, respecting our need for privacy, half-drew the curtain so we could be alone. And then I told her stories about our life together.

I described sailing up the coast in our boat, anchoring in a creek where the only sound was the lap of water against our dinghy, towed on a rope behind us, and the lonely call of oystercatchers. The sun fell late, and the tide dropped around us, revealing shelves of shining mud where the waterbirds stalked, lifting delicate legs and probing the silt with long beaks. Felixstowe docks cast an orange bloom in the sky behind us. Landwards we could see no lights at all. When evening came the sky darkened against a fringe of grass and reeds. I described everything: the hurricane lamp glowing in the cabin; the call of sea birds across the mudflats. I described the stars when we went into the cockpit last thing at night, and our riding light reflected in the oily water.

I described an evening taking the bus to Brixton to see a film at the Ritzy; Brixton market afterwards; the bus home. A day in France, lunch on the terrace, and a walk in the afternoon. A party at home, friends' faces around the table in candlelight. Coming home from a show over Waterloo Bridge, with lights shining from tower blocks and the tide slipping under the arches. They were memories polished and crafted, tidied in the way one might pull weeds from a flowerbed to let the plants grow. The stories were a record of our life's blissful happiness; of our astonishing luck. Rings on a bed of velvet; jewels brought out not for every day, but for a special occasion. It was our taking stock, though we didn't yet know it, of the treasure we had amassed together. We had carved our love into so many days, like lovers cutting their initials in the bark of a tree. There was no greed in it, just a deep-rooted sense of our good fortune.

My voice grew tired. Sometimes I thought Nicola was asleep but, if I stopped, her eyes would open again. I'd carry on: water bubbling in our boat's wake; a pile of artichokes on a market stall in France. It was our life idealised, I suppose; but there was no fiction in it, just a removal of grit, as an archaeologist might dust earth from a long-buried statue, or a restorer swab layers of varnish from a painting until its colours glowed. In stories, sitting beside Nicola's bed, we could travel anywhere. The world was going wrong outside; we were a fortnight away from the Brexit vote. It made no difference to us. In our lost world, the valley to which we'd escaped, nothing outside mattered.

Nicola would be asleep by eight, usually. I went home to cook supper for Martha and Joe. We never stayed up long. I liked to visit Nicola before work, to see how the night had gone. She was always livelier in the mornings, though I couldn't stay more than half an hour – my early visits were a matron's dispensation that I didn't want to abuse. On my way back down the steps I'd call Anne to tell her how Nicola had slept and what the nurse had said.

Anne always wanted more, of course; we both did. We wanted someone to throw us the lifeline of comfort: *She's doing really well, getting on faster than we expected. She'll be up in a fortnight* … It didn't happen. The figures winking on her monitor stayed obstinately the same. The machine was still doing most of her breathing for her.

A microbiologist visited, trying to hunt down the infection that, so her markers indicated, was still there in Nicola's blood. They'd given her the strongest antibiotic they had – 'Domestos,' they joked. It wasn't strong enough. They tried to wean her off steroids, too: one doctor thought the immune reaction over. But she lurched backwards and we had three bad days when she was weak and confused.

They wheeled her off for a scan, then the consultant called us into his office.

'I'm afraid I have to warn you how serious the situation is.'

Joe was beside me, Martha at home. I called Anne afterwards. Nicola's lungs were worse than ever. They were telling us, again, that they thought she might die. They wanted to raise her sedation, put her to sleep so her lungs could recover. We agreed. Stooping to kiss Nicola's forehead, I tried to explain. She understood already. For the second time, I felt as if I might be saying goodbye, but couldn't say so. Martha arrived. We held Nicola's hands as they turned up the sedatives. I could feel grief choking inside me like a weed growing through the foundations of a building. We couldn't lose her; Nicola was everything, to all of us. Her eyes were closed and her mouth fell slack. Air hissed in her tube.

'Rest may help,' the doctor said. 'It may help.'

With each decline, each recovery, the three of us felt like steel tempered. Stressed and relaxed; heated, then plunged into the coldest water. I don't know whether it strengthened or fatigued us. Somehow life went on. We shopped, cooked; I went to work. Martha finished her exams. Joe's jet lag faded.

Nicola lay with her eyes closed, as if we were just her dream, everything around her, my face, conjured into existence behind her flickering eyelids. It was June, by now, the 8th or 9th. We sat by her bed; shuffled our chairs around when the nurse needed to reach a screen or swap a syringe. The numbers winked endlessly: blood pressure, oxygen. On the other side of the bed were the racks of drugs that kept her body stable, floating in the quiet dark while her bruised lungs healed, while the oxygen filled her tired, poisoned blood. There was nothing to say or do. Sometimes we talked. At others, I was alone with her. We kept the door half-closed. Outside, voices murmured. In the room there was nothing between us, now, but memories. Her whiteboard lay on the trolley, the pens in rows, lidded. To talk felt like stirring darkness. Sometimes when she was asleep I'd watch her face; the line of her hair, her wide, closed mouth; or sometimes wake up and find her watching me. But she was further away, now, than sleep; a spaceship voyaging away from the earth, our signals to her becoming ever fainter.

When Nicola was gone, five months after this, we held a celebration at the Roundhouse. Nicola's friend and boss Marcus had offered it – he wanted to help. They put a plaque on one of the columns. Everything that happens there now – bands, theatre, circus, or kids performing poetry – all that energy, happens under an iron plaque with Nicola's name on it. It's better than a gravestone.

For the celebration we invited everyone we could think of, who'd feel her absence and want to mark it. Family and friends poured into the studio where Joe spoke first. He was brilliant: upright and brave, honest, strong. Martha didn't want to speak, then, but I said a few words, then we drank to Nicola. Upstairs, others were already arriving. They flooded up the great staircase, jammed the landing at the top, talking non-stop – Nicola would have loved to hear them talking. Inside, the Roundhouse crew had set up lights. The dome was filled with music. We'd made a playlist of every song she loved: the tracks she'd danced to at Oxford, our favourite tunes from when we first went out, Nina Simone, BB King; the music that had tied us together as a family, the Felice Brothers, The Low Anthem; bands she'd discovered at the Roundhouse, songs Martha and Joe had introduced us to. We had known, of course, how much Nicola was valued in her world, but not how many would flow into the Roundhouse, filling it with talk and love.

Nicola's friend David spoke first – about talking, the root of art. The Roundhouse choir sang, beautifully. Two poets spoke. Marcus, restraining tears, captured the essence of what everyone was feeling; that under that giant dome where art was made, and joy felt, Nicola was there, was with us still.

Afterwards we stood exhausted at the door, Martha, Joe and I, saying goodbye. We took the tube home with friends.

Nicola would have hated grief. Sitting here now, on our last morning in Rome, I can feel it still, grief's river tugging at my knees.

Nicola's breathing recovered, slowly recovered. Her numbers crept upwards again. We were with her when she opened her eyes, drowsily, and looked at me. She seemed unfocused; I don't know what she saw. She squeezed my hand.

'You've done so well,' the nurse said.

She looked so tired, but in another day she was writing again, and looking around. They took another scan. It showed no change, but no deterioration either.

'From a transplant point of view,' the consultant said, 'she's doing OK.'

Like reeling in a kite, we pulled her back to us. It proved again how strong Nicola was. She could walk along death's riverbank, trail her foot in the water, and still come back.

Another day and she had made up the lost ground. She smiled, raised her eyebrows. *Notebooks*, she wrote on the whiteboard. I brought in spiral-bound notebooks and a pen. She scribbled busily, covering page after page. I had to buy more. She chatted, via her notebooks, with the nurses. One of them was getting married. Nicola wanted to know more. Her thirst for life was greater than ever; she sucked it in just as her lungs sucked in oxygen, greedy for air. With the tip of her pen she directed where she wanted photographs moved to.

The staff were pleased. They stood around her bed, tired. Nicola wrote busily, *You should be taking proper breaks.* When I went out onto the steps each morning, to call Anne, I had to temper her enthusiasm. There was still a long way to go, I said. It was amazing how she had bounced back but she wasn't out of danger. I felt as if I was taking treats away from a child. Nicola texted me for the first time in days. I texted hearts, she texted back, *x10000000000.*

All the same, I could tell how tired she was. And for the first time since her lungs started to fail, for the first time in our whole year-long journey, Nicola showed signs of anxiety. Sometimes, when I wasn't there, she panicked. It made her breathing worse; then they had to switch up the oxygen. I was more frightened by her loss of confidence than anything: Nicola had been so strong since the first afternoon, that awful moment, when we met on the corner of Wincott Street after the doctor's call.

Reason didn't help. I said, 'You're being so well looked after. There are nurses and doctors all around you. Think of something soothing. Think of Martha and Joe.'

I knew it was no use; you can't reach fear. And Nicola was confused, baffled by Fentanyl and the other drugs they poured into her, trying to keep her alive. Perhaps the antibiotics, a thick sediment clogging her blood, contributed to it as well; and the claustrophobia of bed, unmoving; the machines seen from the corner of her eye; the conversations outside, half-heard; the doctors' unreadable expressions as they scanned her notes; and, most of all, the tube gripping her throat, squeezing her neck. Of course she panicked.

Are you coming to see me this afternoon? she texted; then followed it up, seconds later, with question marks. We agreed a system. I drew a chart on a laminated board, a column for each day. At the top I wrote the name of the nurse looking after her. That helped her, blurrily, to keep track of time. I wrote who would come to see her and when. I'd agreed with work to go to the hospital Monday, Wednesday and Friday. Anne visited on the other afternoons. Nicola looked at the chart, nodded as far as the tube allowed her. It was a structure of sorts.

She texted, *Battery running v low but good morning and I love you even more today than I have in the last 28 years. Xxxxx.* I didn't know if she meant her phone's battery, or her own. I texted back, *My sweet sweet darling I always told you I'd love you more and more and I do.*

Dear All, I wrote to friends, almost the last message I'd send them,

> I thought you'd want an update, and lots of you have
> been asking, so it's good to be able to say that things

are looking a lot better now than a fortnight ago. We're still facing a long recovery process, with quite a stretch in Intensive Care while Nicola stays on the ventilator. And, of course, there are still risks of further infection etc. But she's back with us, unsedated, feeling very positive & upbeat (as you would expect), and busily scribbling notes on a paper pad, while trying to catch up with all the Intensive Care Unit nurses' gossip. Full recovery is still in our sights, however far off. The haematology doctors are very upbeat about the transplant.

Reading it now, I can hear the note of false cheer in it, almost of desperation. But we didn't despair. We were still clinging to hope.

I arranged for the Transplant Unit's counsellor, whom Nicola had met before, to come and see us both. He listened. I hated talking on Nicola's behalf – I kept apologising, kept checking with her to see if I'd expressed things the way she wanted. Nicola was the patient; she was the one who needed his help. Tired, she wrote on a pad, nodded, listened.

The next morning she texted, asking me to come. It was a muddled message. I wasn't sure if she meant to come straightaway, or was confused about what time I'd be there at the end of the day. And by now I was feeling the strain myself. I wondered if I should give up work and just look after Nicola, but she would hate that – or so, at least, I told myself. And since we were both certain she would recover, we needed to keep our lives intact. I sent a long text back, equally garbled, then called the ward to see how she was, and spoke to her nurse. In the end I stayed at work, worrying whether I was doing the right thing or not. I felt guilty – I still feel guilty. I felt selfish for needing work as a rest from the Frank Stansil Unit. Nicola's recovery could go on for months, I told myself. We had to pace ourselves. The doctors had told us the same thing.

Nicola texted back, *All good. Come when you can.* It still didn't feel right. For the first time in her year of illness, I felt I wasn't standing shoulder-to-shoulder beside her, but two paces behind, looking at her – as if I couldn't keep up. We talked when I reached the ward. I talked, she wrote. I suggested leaving my job. *Of course not*, she wrote firmly. *What you're saying is right.* But it still didn't feel right. What choice did she have but to agree with me? All the same, I knew that I didn't have the strength to be there every minute, as she was.

Nicola was stronger next day, busy with texts. I had a meeting in Kent. I texted, *Sitting in Tunbridge Wells Council meeting. I'd rather be in Intensive Care.* She texted hearts.

The week's consultant was brusque but encouraging. She said, 'In my view, we're now in a recovery pattern.'

She was keen to get Nicola up. It took a whole team of nurses to manoeuvre her onto a special chair. She didn't want them to put her back to bed until I reached the hospital to see her. I cycled as fast as I could, arrived just in time to see her perched there, queen on a throne, with Joe beside her. He and I went for a cup of tea while they manhandled her back into bed.

'For her,' the nurse said, 'that'll be the equivalent of running a marathon. She'll be exhausted tomorrow.'

So she was, but pleased with herself. She did some breathing exercises. She was weaker, perhaps, than the doctors had expected; another scan was ordered. She texted, *I'm feeling mentally much better but exhausted.*

The next day, Friday, was the morning after Brexit. I went into the office and found colleagues sitting in stunned silence. Many came from elsewhere in Europe; their world had caved in. I wanted to hurry to the ward and be with Nicola. When I got there, early afternoon, the nurses were standing by her door.

They greeted me as usual – nothing had changed – but when I went in, I knew something was wrong. Nicola seemed drowsier than before, listless.

I mentioned it to a nurse, who frowned.

'Her stats haven't changed. I'll get a doctor.'

The doctor examined her but found nothing new. Nicola's eyes were closed.

'We'll keep an eye on her,' he said.

Looking through texts now I can see the end coming. The blue texts on the right of the printout are mine; hers, in grey, are on the left. Reading through them, I can see the signs leading towards the end: *Battery running low ... exhausted ...* The next morning, Saturday, I texted, *Hello?* The page is empty after that. Nicola never replied.

When I arrived at the hospital that morning she was half-asleep. A new consultant was there, a burly man, Italian. He looked concerned: the oxygen in Nicola's blood was dropping. I sat at the end of her bed, trying not to watch the figures decline. Each time the nurse stepped forward to increase the flow, and I heard the whistle of gas in the line, it felt like a small defeat, another withdrawal; a defensive line abandoned. Martha and Joe arrived. Nicola's eyes fluttered. When she tried to write on her pad, the writing wasn't hers: it was weak, shapeless. I look at it again sometimes now, leafing through the pages of the notebooks I've kept. As the pages turn, the well-formed words begin to melt. By the end she could only manage a scrawl.

I remember taking the pen out of her hand when she was too tired to go on. Her head fell sideways. I noticed a twitch in her face. Nothing, until then, had come so close to breaking my heart. She was trying to grin at us, but couldn't. Her cheeks twitched, not quite under control. Her mouth widened, and then fell slack again.

As the day went on, the doctors grew more and more worried. Never giving up, they ordered another scan. We wheeled Nicola through corridors, and watched through a window as they slid her into the scanner. The doctors were looking for some sign her infection was diminishing or that the fluid drowning her lungs was drying.

It wasn't.

The consultant said, 'We're going to take control of her breathing again.'

But it wasn't just that: Nicola's kidneys were tiring from the volume of fluid they pumped out of her, trying to dry her lungs. She was half-asleep by now.

A nurse had explained: 'As carbon dioxide builds up in her blood, it will make her drowsy.'

Nicola never knew she was going to die. The week before, we'd told the doctors we no longer wanted to talk to them in the office – we wanted to talk by Nicola's bed, where she could hear. Now, though, the consultant led us into his room. It must have been Saturday afternoon.

He said, 'Her condition is very serious.'

I tried to keep my head up. Joe and Martha were with me. 'We understand.'

'We need to put her on kidney dialysis,' he explained. But it wasn't the detail of her medical condition that mattered, it was the expression on his face.

Another machine was wheeled to Nicola's bedside. We sat on chairs outside while they wired it up, then watched wheels spin, cleansing her blood, as if the sickness could be wrung from it to leave her limp but well.

'We'll let her sleep,' one of the doctors said. 'It helped before.'

It had – sleep had let her recover, and she'd woken better. The nurse said, 'Are you ready now?'

They increased the sedative. Nicola was so drowsy already that she could hardly feel us take her hands. Weakly she squeezed my fingers. I was trying not to cry. Her cheeks twitched, sketching her marvellous smile, then giving up, exhausted. Her eyes closed.

I put one arm round Martha's shoulders as we left the room. Joe was very quiet.

Nicola was like that for a day, or perhaps a bit more. Waking at night, I checked my phone for messages, then cycled to the hospital as early as I could. No change. But on Monday morning, her numbers were lower still. The consultant was already standing by her door, surrounded by nurses and the matron.

His face said everything; he didn't need to speak.

I called Martha and Joe, and Anne. I said, 'It's probably time you should come and see her.'

In the office the consultant asked whether we wanted to let her go slowly, or whether they should switch off the machines. There was no more hope, he said. Martha and Joe sat either side of me.

I looked at Martha and Joe for confirmation, then said, 'Just give us time to say goodbye. Then let her go.'

Anne and Peter arrived. We left them alone with her. Then we went in ourselves. Martha and Joe, her children, Nicola … the four of us had been a unit for so long. Now we were together for the last time.

When Martha and Joe went out, I stood with her for a while myself, then said to the nurse, 'We're ready.'

She closed the door. It was a simple enough thing; they just turned off the machines that had been keeping Nicola alive, tirelessly, for the last five weeks. I held her hand; she didn't hold mine. One by one the nurse switched off monitors, closed syringes. The room fell silent. I hadn't realised how much noise it made, life. Now everything was quiet. It was just Nicola and me. I told her how much I loved her, but I was really only telling myself. I traced my finger along the line where her hair had fallen. I touched the mouth I'd kissed so often. The line of her jaw, her ear – I wanted to imprint them forever on my eyes, so I could always see her. There was so much that hadn't changed – her foot under the sheet, her fingers squeezed between my own. So much of her was well. I reached down to kiss her forehead. It was like pressing my lips to ivory. The pain welling up inside me was a pressure almost intolerable. We had been so happy together, so lucky in each other. We had said everything, but there was still so much more to say.

The nurse stood at the half-open door. 'She's gone.'

She quietly switched off the last monitors. Took away the tube so her neck was free. My love lay on the pillow, gone. Switched off, all the memories in her head, of me and her children, of the time before me; a whole life of thoughts and dreams, of knowledge, of people – erased. Our loneliness was complete.

Martha and Joe came back in. None of us wanted to stay in the room long; Nicola was no longer there. I had a moment of not wanting to leave the body I'd so loved, but it was only a foolish impulse. She wasn't there; we were alone. We walked out of the ward. Anne and Peter had already left. Down in the street it was sunny.

One of us said, 'Let's go to Greenwich.'

It felt as if we'd known all along that Nicola would die, though we'd always expected life. It feels, now, as if I've never left the room she died in; as if I'm standing there, still, by her bedside, touching her cheek. I don't know that I will ever leave. We drove to Greenwich. Wind stirred the trees; the river flowed beneath us. We talked about Nicola, but about other things too. Back home, later, I emailed friends:

I'm so sorry to do this by email, but can't face so many calls.

I'm afraid that Nicola was hit by another deterioration at the weekend. This time she was too weak to sustain it. We're terribly sad to have to tell you that she died earlier today, completely peacefully. Martha, Joe and I were with her.

The three of us want you all to know that we're going to cope with this the way Nicola would. We don't want gloom. We want to keep remembering how wonderful she is; and looking ahead and staying positive, as she always did.

Epilogue

The weekend after Nicola died we held a party for her in our garden. We only invited the people we loved most. Some were probably missed – there was nothing organised about it. Before Nicola fell ill we'd been planning a joint celebration of our twenty-fifth wedding anniversary, Joe's eighteenth birthday, and Nicola's fiftieth. I'd bought cheap tents on eBay. Now we set them up, prising open boxes that had stood abandoned in the basement for twelve months. Martha and Joe draped coloured lights across the lawn.

As the doorbell rang, our friends came in with plates of food. Foxgloves nodded in the darkening flowerbeds. Music played in the kitchen, a playlist we'd put together of all the songs Nicola had ever loved and danced to. Anne and Peter came too, and I realised then how much of our lives had been founded on theirs: their values and principles, their love for people and for art. At the party, Anne had tears in her eyes but didn't give in to them; she was too brave for that. Peter talked. They didn't stay long.

I knew early on that I needed to write this story. I said at the start it wasn't sad, and I still mean that. Nicola's illness was the most terrible year of our life together but it contained the purest moments of love we ever shared. Nicola was never more herself. Her sweetness, her humour, her love and intelligence were honed by sickness to their purest and final shape. She never loved the people around her more. She never valued so clearly what the world offered, or what she had given it. We saw far. And we realised our story, which had, like all stories, to end someday, was the happiest we could ever have hoped for.

Since she died, since the day when we went up to Greenwich, we've been trying to live without her.

The year before she fell ill Nicola put on Monteverdi's *L'Orfeo*, in partnership with the Royal Opera House. We never dreamed that she one day would be Eurydice and that I would have to follow her, searching for Hades' gates. The other night I had a dream that she'd been seen on an island

and I found myself there. I asked a man on the quayside where she might be. He said she'd gone inland, but she wasn't on the island anymore.

'How could she have left the island,' I asked, 'if she went inland?'

He looked at me and said, 'How did you get here yourself?'

I couldn't answer. I long to have the dream again. Within it, I believed there was a chance I really could find Nicola and bring her back.

People tell me I'm doing well, but I know there's something wrong with me. I snap at them; I'm impatient; I disagree. There's a surliness in me that feels as alien as a cancer, a dog padding at my side. There's a darkness on the horizon behind me. There's a black sea in front of me, and with every step I take, its waters rise higher about my legs.

Sometimes I just want to stay still. To sit in a chair with my eyes closed, to silence phones and computers, to stop everything moving and stay motionless, as if I had to hold myself rigid to staunch a flow of blood. But I don't stay still – I go out, I work. It seems best to do things, frenetically if need be, rather than let silence fall.

And we've done a lot in the time since Nicola died.

In October, four months afterwards, Martha, Joe and I went to Buckingham Palace to collect her OBE. We worried the occasion would be stuffy, but it was perfectly managed, with good humour and a welcome for the excited families, none of us grand, who gathered in the courtyard beforehand. Everyone was happy to be there; no one was made to feel ill at ease. Standing in the wings during the presentation, I listened to the military band playing light hits on the balcony and realised they were halfway through 'Stairway to Heaven'. 'Mamma Mia!' followed. Nicola would have wept with laughter. We have a photograph of the three of us outside, holding Nicola's OBE in a leather case, the sun shining. Afterwards Anne and Peter took us out to lunch.

On our walks at Pin Mill, Nicola and I talked about the places that meant most to us – London and Suffolk, Rome, the Peloponnese and south-west France. We've been back to all of them in the months since she died. Call it a pilgrimage, if you like. I suppose I wanted to visit them for the same reason Nicola and I always returned: to keep them alive by constant renewal, like Australians tracking songlines to keep a bush in flower, a spring flowing, a rock balanced on a cliff.

I'm in France now, at Easter, as I write this epilogue. France is where we fell in love, and where our life together unfolded; it was the place we brought up our children. Driving past each bend in the road, each tree, I'm passing memories of almost thirty years together. Nicola is with me at every age: twenty years old, still carrying puppy fat, and something gauche that soon dusted away, like mildew off a leaf; a mother of two babies, sterilising jars; at the summit of her poise, two years ago; or hunched in a chaise longue, wearing a headscarf.

Remembering her is like watching my own soul grow old. She was my soul's vessel, freighting it across oceans. Without her I feel a phantom in this tough countryside. The trees are older than me, stronger and more rooted. Even the birds seem more vivid. I feel invisible, as if no one will be aware of me when I stop on a hill, at a point where we once stopped together. Then, our voices might have been heard in the farm below, our footsteps sniffed by a dog; or threads from our coats built into a jay's nest. Today I make no sound, leave no mark. This isn't my place anymore. I came here with Nicola; without her I can only wander through it, unresting. It feels as if I'm haunting my own past life.

Out here a couple of months ago, I drove past the house where we used to live. My wheels splashed through puddles; it had rained. The water in those puddles fell twenty years ago; Nicola was beside me. In my half-state, I can fold time aside like layers of curtain, or like dust sheets pleated into a trunk to enfold a dress still faintly perfumed. Time seems as thin as paper, and as brittle, crumbling to dust as my hand passes through it; or as my eye sweeps a hillside where we walked, once, the children in carriers on our backs. I can hear the crunch of gravel under our wheels as we turn onto the drive, tired from twelve hours' journey; our headlights sweep a patch of wall, a rose cut back for winter, and the locked door. They are all still there, those moments, inaccessible to the living, but visible to me in my waking sleep.

Nicola rests gently on the pillow next to me when I wake up; I can almost hear her breath. Then, when I sit up, she is gone, abruptly gone, and the earth's weight falls heavily around me; roofs pressing down towards earth, the trees bowing under their leaves' weight, and the clouds freighted with lead. In moments like this I understand death's permanence. I glimpse Nicola; but she isn't coming back. Reality is final, after all: final without appeal.

I know, suddenly and far too young, what old people know: how to live life looking only backwards; to survey it from a hill with the sea at your back and nowhere further to go but a path ending in couch-grass. How to pick out a hill in the distance, looking back, and remember the sweat beading our foreheads as we climbed it, the weight of our packs. Or to identify, hidden among trees, a bridge, a ford, a village where we stopped; a lake rimmed with ice; the house where our child was born.

But memories carry no taste of life, just ash. No one warned Nicola and me that our journey was reaching its end.

We thought there were miles still to travel, our footsteps slowing gradually together. We thought, perfectly timed, we'd reach the final crest together just as our strength failed; lie down in the grass together, fall asleep with the sound of curlews presaging the sea.

Instead, I'm here alone: strong, healthy enough, and stupidly alive. I don't know what to do. Sit on a bench. Revolve memories whose lines are already blurred from over-use, like charms fingered too often. I can set in motion a whole pageant of memory, clownish figures spinning along memory's prescribed grooves, endlessly repeating the same motions, but they never comfort me. Life is only worth anything as each moment conjures itself into being. What's left behind is just the worm's cast, the snake's sloughed-off skin; life's refuse and detritus; a slag-hill of memories that we pile up around us, all mineral value mined from it to leave raw clay.

In some ways what's happened is a terrifying acceleration towards old age, when everything I love will be in the past.

And the world is already changing around me, although I don't want it to. The trees are growing up around the house. There's a sapling sprouting by the terrace. About the time Nicola went in for her transplant I stubbed my toe, a blood blister under the nail. I've watched it slowly growing out. Soon I'll cut it off at the nail and that moment will be gone. The time when Nicola was still alive is growing out, through my nails, my hair. I can't stop myself changing, or hold myself in the time she knew. I can't wrestle the sun or clamp the earth in its tracks. It rolls me away like a wheel, and Nicola dwindles behind me, left at the roadside.

Orpheus made his way to the Underworld to bring his lover back again. I don't know what to make of the story of Pluto's bargain: that he could lead her back to life so long as he never looked back. I understand better the image of him walking the woods, singing of Eurydice. A week ago, Martha, Joe and I buried Nicola's ashes here, and planted a tree. This isn't a sad place – Nicola was never a sad person. She was more at home in the world than anyone I ever met. She had judgement in the truest sense. I don't just mean her aesthetic taste, exquisite though that was, but her instinct about things that should be done, and things that were wrong, or that shouldn't be worried about. She lived life more accurately than anyone I ever knew, placing her footsteps with the grace of a dancer through friendship, work, love, parenthood. Life buoyed her up. She was at home in it as a dolphin in water, playfully; at home in it as she was in her own skin. Her death came far too early for Martha and Joe, and for me, but that gap will close as the rest of us grow old, and we come nearer to her.

I long to be nearer to her. Outside the door I can see the place where her ashes lie, and beyond it the forests and hills. I know that it can never be like this, because loss is final, but I wish I could find her again. I wish I had never looked back. I wish I could be there now, with her hand in mine and the smell of earth around us, walking in the trees' shadow.

Patrick Dillon
27 June 2017

Acknowledgements

This book has been made possible by some wonderful, kind and sensitive support. Andrew Lownie, my agent for twenty years, and a friend of Nicola's as well, took it under his wing with exactly the right combination of tact and thoughtfulness, and removed all pressure from me. I could not be more grateful to him. Robyn Drury, at Ebury, responded to the book straightaway. She seemed to understand instinctively why I needed to write it, and what I wanted to say. Robyn's wisdom and intuition as an editor has been invaluable, and perfectly judged. Claire Scott, Diana Riley and the rest of the Ebury team have been ceaselessly kind, patient and sensitive in shepherding it to publication. I am truly grateful to all of them.

I am grateful to the friends who read a manuscript that can only have been painful in recalling a year that left them, too, bereft. Their love and support sustained Nicola through illness. They've carried me, Martha and Joe through the time since she died.

Finally, and most of all, I want to thank Martha and Joe. This book describes a year that devastated us, changed us, and brought us closer together. They were the first to read the manuscript; without their support I would not have published it. *A Moment of Grace* is for them, with infinite love.

The Nicola Thorold Fund

Nicola's work at the Roundhouse still goes on. After she died, we set up the Nicola Thorold Fund in her memory. The Roundhouse's brilliant mission is to help young people through the arts. We wanted to go on being part of it. You can support it too, and find out more about it, at http://www.roundhouse.org.uk/about-us/support-our-work/the-nicola-thorold-fund/.